AIDS: WHAT THE DISCOVERERS
OF HIV NEVER ADMITTED

Lawrence Broxmeyer, M.D.

AIDS: WHAT THE DISCOVERERS OF HIV NEVER ADMITTED

COPYRIGHT: US LIBRARY OF CONGRESS

Third Edition

Published by
New Century Press
1055 Bay Boulevard, Suite C
Chula Vista, CA 91911
(800) 519–2465
(619) 476–7400
www.newcenturypress.com
sales@newcenturypress.com
Cover Design by New Century Press

ISBN 1-890035-29-7

Other titles by Lawrence Broxmeyer, M.D.
Parkinson's Disease-Another Look
www.parkinsonsdiseaseanotherlook.com

To Alvia:

A breath of fresh air,

a free spirit,

in a

corrupt and contaminated world

CONTENTS

FORWARD iii

PROLOGUE.. v

1/ EPIDEMIC 1

2/ CANCER STRUGGLES.................................... 5

3/ SHYH-CHING LO.. 9

4/ IN THE SEMEN OF MAN 13

5/ CATS.. 21

6/ TRAGIC COST OF PREMATURE CONSENSUS........ 25

7/ THE RACE 27

8/ INVISIBLE VIRUS....................................... 32

9/ SMOKE AND MIRRORS................................ 35

10/ AMBIGUOUS SLAUGHTER............................ 39

11/ VIRAL MIRAGE 45

12/ LUCKY 49

REFERENCES.. 57

INDEX 79

FORWARD

I did not write this book with any particular intent other than to set the record straight. Sometime in 1991, when I was splitting time treating AIDS patients with research endeavors with colleagues in San Francisco and Nebraska, I got a call from Genivive Clavruel of Project Win on behalf of Luc Montagnier, discoverer of HIV.

She had received my AIDS research proposal under confidentiality agreement and forwarded a copy to Montagnier. Yes, she wanted to talk about it.

But about half–way through the conversation, her voice changed, steadily diminishing to almost a whisper.

"Your paper is not as unique an idea as you led me to believe," she said before her voice became an undertone. "Dr. Montagnier also suspects this organism causes AIDS."

"Causes it?"

"Yes."

I felt only disbelief. Montagnier was said to have suspected mycoplasma as a co–factor to HIV at one time in AIDS. But what I sent her was a paper regarding the laboratory protocol to cure AIDS in animals through the destruction of virulent, drug-resistant AIDS TB and avian or fowl TB by the use of phages–viruses found inside bacteria. This paper claimed that HIV did not cause AIDS throughout.

Clavruel was on a roll. Fully realizing her shock value, she abruptly switched current. "What do you want?"

"Just what I said from day one, a collaboration with Montagnier."

"At Pasteur?"

FORWARD
L. Broxmeyer, M.D.

"Why, yes."

"Then I'll ask him for some laboratory space and get back to you."

She never did.

That call ended as abruptly as it had begun. But the questions it raised did not.

If Montagnier really thought AIDS was caused by mycobacteria, such as TB and fowl tuberculosis, then why did he not come out publicly to a world already convinced that his HIV caused AIDS? Was he on a fishing expedition?

Or did he really believe that tuberculosis and fowl tuberculosis were possibly behind AIDS? Whatever the reason, the world and myself were owed an explanation.

But that explanation never came until further research and time made it clear.

Montagnier was already invested in HIV up to his neck with or without his mycoplasma co-factor, which got him into much trouble with his HIV advocates. He could not jump ship in midstream. Someone else would have to present the issue; this book is about that issue.

LB

PROLOGUE

UNIVERSITY OF LIVERPOOL
LIVERPOOL, ENGLAND
1988

The results were disquieting. Researchers at the University of Liverpool, England, in 1988, had found a retrovirus in 97% of the women they tested for breast cancer. (Al-Sumidaie, 1988)

Did this finding mean that breast cancer was also caused by a retrovirus? Certainly not. Al-Sumidaie knew very well as a viral researcher that he could take cells from a patient's body and coax out a lot of harmless retroviruses to which a patient had been exposed. When in the retroviral business, you detected retroviruses and over the years it had been done in multiple sclerosis, sarcomas and leukemias. Yet little more evidence than Al-Sumidaie now had in front of him was available when the HIV retrovirus was called the probable cause of AIDS.

1/ EPIDEMIC

<u>MANHATTAN</u>
<u>1979</u>

By 1979, doctors in Manhattan began to notice a strange new disease killing what had been up to then healthy gay men. As reports mounted, the Centers for Disease Control (CDC) was forced to circulate similar notices of homosexual men in New York and Los Angeles with a weakened immune system dying from heretofore rare causes. (MMWR, 1981) Unnoticed was an earlier raise in the New York infection rate for tuberculosis which, from the onset, the new epidemic emulated.

From its conception AIDS was a nightmare of anguished victims, washed with wave after wave of terrible disease, whose physicians, like so many medical priests, helplessly watched them die. U.S. Coastal hospitals in San Francisco, New York and Los Angeles soon turned into war zones.

Rare diseases like *Pneumocystis carinii,* tiny one-celled protozoa, filled gay lungs to the point of suffocation and requests for pentamidine aerosols trickled and then poured into the CDC.

Another uncommon killer, Kaposi's Sarcoma (KS), became the most common form of AIDS cancer.

Nor was it only gays at risk. Drug addicts sharing needles and hemophiliacs, given pooled clotting factor VIII from blood, so they would not bleed to death, soon became prey, again developing Kaposi's sarcoma and *pneumocystis* pneumonia. America's entire blood supply was in jeopardy, for by the early 1980's, gay and bisexual men accounted for 1 of 4 American blood donors.

AIDS throttled the immune system, in some cases shutting it down, and the primary site of attack always

AIDS: WHAT THE DISCOVERERS
OF HIV NEVER ADMITTED

seemed traceable to the body's T-cells: white blood cell lymphocytes which held the body's invaders at bay.

By 1977 much evidence indicated that the basis of cellular immunity was tied in with T-cells lymphocytes – colorless, motile, cellular elements of lymph. Chief in importance among these was the T-helper or CD4 lymphocyte, which fought infection. It soon became apparent that in AIDS CD4 cells were either severely depleted or, they fell off the blood map altogether.

Without delay, the same virologists who for decades had failed miserably to find a viral cause for cancer, pounced on AIDS, dismissing any possibility other than a virus: ignoring that it could just as easily be either one or a combination of older microbes presenting in an all-new way.

Virologists initially told physicians to pass on the word that Cytomegalovirus (MMWR, 1981) caused AIDS. Doctors dutifully obeyed, not fully realizing that all people, with time, are infected with Cytomegalovirus.

Epidemiologist-retrovirologist Donald Francis, who would direct laboratory efforts for AIDS at the CDC, and was also Assistant Director of the CDC's Division of Viral Diseases, had his own peculiar theory which he shared with epidemiologist James Curran, eventual director of AIDS research at CDC: combine hepatitis with feline leukemia in cats – a retrovirus on which Francis wrote his doctorate and you had Kaposi's and the opportunistic infections seen in AIDS. Or maybe, just maybe, it was a retrovirus similar to the cat retrovirus alone that was solely responsible. Curran and Francis had worked together years ago developing the Hepatitis B vaccine.

Francis, one of the few at CDC who had actively wiped out smallpox worldwide, was considered an expert on both epidemics and the feline leukemic virus. He would now combine his fields of expertise and quickly conclude that AIDS was cat leukemia in people. It was an impulsive long shot and by most treated as such, at least initially.

____

2/ CANCER STRUGGLES

<u>AMERICA</u>
<u>TURN OF THE CENTURY</u>

The history of retroviruses mirrored cancer research. By the turn of the twentieth century American medicine had come to the conclusion that it was not a matter of whether infectious disease caused cancer, but which one. Incredibly, just 20 years before, the germ theory of disease, ignored by organized medicine for 150 years, had finally been accepted. Robert Koch, discoverer of the cause of tuberculosis, had seen to that. But as the "Father of Bacteriology" and perhaps the greatest physician that ever lived, when Koch presented his Berlin paper his immediate problem was in convincing the German medical establishment that TB was not a "virus".

Under this backdrop and in 1904, Ellermann and Bang, searching for an infectious bacterial cause for chicken leukemia (Ellermann & Bang, 1908), succeeded in its transfer from one fowl to another by injecting cell-free tissue infiltrates. They sought a bacteria, but simply because it passed through a filter, the responsible agent was assumed to be a virus.

That same year, the first lentivirus, related to HIV, was isolated as a filterable equine infectious agent by Valle and Carre at the Pasteur Institute. (Valle, 1904) Yet Roux, an authority on 'invisible microbes' at the time, shrugged off Valle and Carre's finding as no more than "small bacteria". (Roux, 1903)

Most authorities now realize that there are some viruses almost as large as bacteria and some bacteria as small as viruses, forms of which can easily pass through filters. This realization has been disputed by HIV enthusiasts Francis, Curran & Essex when they mentioned, "since the infectious agent had obviously passed through a filter, it had to be a virus". (Francis, Curran & Essex, 1983)

It did not.

Peyton Rous was credited with the discovery and isolation of the first retrovirus. By 1911, Rous wanted to know why if one chicken got cancer, others followed. (Rous, 1911) Rous, who reproduced the tumor at will in Plymouth Rock fowls, favored a bacterial cause over a filterable virus. However, it was a question that he never definitely answered.

By 1933 Shope reported a viral tumor in cottontail rabbits. Bittner reported on a milk-born mouse breast cancer attributed to still another virus. (Bittner, 1936)

In the 1950s, and with the advent of the electron microscope, particles later questionably ascribed to retroviruses were readily being detected. As a result, and at a time when established medicine had about-faced and was now firmly set against an infectious cause for cancer, two controversial minority camps splintered from mainstream, each diametrically opposed.

There were the virologists, who claimed that cancer was viral, and another group, which did careful, peer-reviewed research at the height of U.S. Post-World War II technology, demonstrating that the retroviruses in Rous, Bittner and Shope tumors were actually mycobacterial-like bacteria of the *Actinomycetales*. (Livingston, 1972)

Tuberculosis-like, these 'viruses' stained with acid-fast dyes; readily passed through a filter, but actually were a class of bacteria having many of the characteristics of the mycobacteria such as tuberculosis.

This work, spearheaded by physician-researcher Virginia Livingston of Rutgers (Livingston, 1970), validated earlier work on the Rous agent as a bacteria. (Duran-Reynals, 1950; Glover & Scott, 1926) Soon others would join.

Chapter 2/ CANCER STRUGGLES
L. Broxmeyer, M.D.

(Alexander Jackson, 1954; Diller, 1970; Seibert & Feldman, 1970)

Livingston's network questioned the very existence of retroviruses and the retrovirologists did not like it. A scientific life-and-death cancer struggle ensued.

By 1960, biologist turned retrovirologist Howard Temin sought an explanation for his observation as to why retroviruses, composed of RNA, Rous among them, were inhibited by Actinomycin D – an antibiotic and known bacterial DNA inhibitor. Based on this finding, Temin elaborately hypothesized the concept of reverse transcription. But since antibiotics did not affect viruses, Temin's observation regarding Actinomycin D's inhibition of Rous made more sense if Rous was bacterial.

Nevertheless, in reaction to Temin, cancer viral investigators of the '60's and '70's reacted by misinterpreting his non-specific enzyme discovery (reverse transcriptase), which arose primarily as a function of normal cellular healing, for a primary indicator for the newly scrutinized retroviruses – which it was not. And in the 1970's, it was as a direct result of Temin's enzyme that "oncoviruses", purported to cause cancer, suddenly became "retroviruses".

It was to Livingston's solid disadvantage that when Richard Nixon signed his National Cancer Act on December 23, 1971, he unwittingly placed virologist Frank Rauscher as director of the just established National Cancer Program (NCP). With Rauscher at the controls it was only a matter of time before cancer virologists, retrovirologists and immunologists were pushed to the vanguard of "America's War on Cancer". Once entrenched, they would remain at the helm even as, incredibly, their failed cancer attempts now turned towards finding a viral cause for AIDS.

Bacterial L-forms, the connecting link between viruses and bacteria, were first described by Klieneberger at England's Lister Institute for which they were named. L-Forms were "cell-wall deficient" because they either had a disruption or lack of a rigid bacterial cell wall. This lack of rigidity allowed them the plasticity to assume many forms (pleomorphic), some of them viral-like but all different from their classical parent and poorly confirmed by ordinary staining. (Klieneberger-Nobel, 1949) Of all the bacteria, L-forms predominate and are crucial to the survival of the mycobacteria whose cell-wall-deficient (CWD) forms escape destruction by the body's immune system. And at the same time CWD forms of the mycobacteria react in ELISA blood tests (Mattman, 1993), similar to the "HIV virus," and can simulate it in everyway.

Some years later, when HIV discoverer Luc Montagnier was interviewed for a French AIDS documentary, filmmaker Djamel Tabi asked how he had isolated HIV. Incredibly, Montagnier's reply was that he did not isolate HIV, he just found something that looked like a retrovirus. (Null, 2000)

Klieneberger, as well as Livingston, also saw parallels between the filterable forms of tuberculosis and "mycoplasmic-like forms" because without intact cell walls they were often mistaken for the virus-like bacteria mycoplasma, which has no cell wall. (Livingston, 1970) The differentiation between mycoplasma and cell-wall-deficient bacteria is difficult at best. (Mattman, 1993)

3/ SHYH-CHING LO

<u>ARMED FORCES INSTITUTE OF PATHOLOGY</u>
<u>WASHINGTON</u>
<u>1989</u>

Dr. Shyh-Ching Lo was a senior scientist at the prestigious, world-renowned Armed Forces Institute of Pathology in Washington. As he watched events unfold and it became obvious that it was going to be dictum that HIV caused AIDS, he just had one problem: whenever he examined someone who had died of AIDS, he could never find HIV, not even a trace of HIV-infected tissue damage. So Lo began his own search for an AIDS cause, which led him to a "virus-like infectious agent". (Lo, 1986) Knowing he was onto something, Shyh-Ching Lo followed his conscience, against the grain of most other scientists, and finally isolated a mycoplasma. And in one study of 24 people with AIDS, he found antibody titers to it in practically every one. (Lo & Dawson, 1989) Shyh-Ching Lo co-published again with Saillard. (Saillard, 1990)

That same year Livingston died and a year later Luc Montagnier, the discoverer of HIV almost got booed off a 1991 San Francisco podium at an International AIDS conference for endorsing Lo's mycoplasma as a necessary co-factor for the AIDS virus to become fatal. (Ostrom, 1991) This "co-factor" theory was, in effect Montagnier's way of admitting that HIV, the virus he had discovered, was not virulent enough in itself to even approach what happened in AIDS.

Montagnier and Lemaitre had done a hornet's nest of an experiment that put HIV advocates on the edge of their chairs. In 1990 they published that cells cultured with "HIV", which normally died, grew well in the presence of two antibiotics, minocycline and doxycycline. (Lemaitre, 1990) Antibiotics do not affect viruses, so it wasn't working against HIV – it was a bacteria. Montagnier decided that that bacteria was probably Lo's mycoplasma. He had done so unaware that the two particular antibiotics he was using also had activity against Livingston's mycobacteria. (Roussel & Igual, 1998; Taska and Urano, 1995; Gupta & Kocher, 1992; Burns & Rohatge, 1990; Tsukamura, 1984)

RUTGERS-PRESBYTERIAN HOSPITAL LABORATORY
FOR THE STUDY OF PROLIFERATIVE DISEASES
BUREAU OF BIOLOGICAL RESEARCH
RUTGERS UNIVERSITY
NEW JERSEY
1950

Livingston associate and prominent Cornell microbiologist Eleanor Alexander-Jackson (1954), a lifelong colleague, had a problem.

As long as she held her reputation as one of the leading tuberculosis experts in the world, American medicine would embrace her, but when she tried to attribute cancer to Livingston's tuberculosis-like germ, it would move to crush her.

Alexander-Jackson, whose advanced mycobacterial staining and culture techniques appeared in a 1944 issue of *Science,* carefully set a trap insured to ensnare virologists. Rous, as a retrovirus, was supposed to be an RNA virus; Alexander-Jackson knew that finding DNA in it would automatically mean that it was bacterial. It was understood that Retroviral DNA should be present only in human or animal cells and nowhere else.

Her paper on the *Ultraviolet Spectrogramic Microscope Studies of Rous Sarcoma Virus Cultured in Cell Free Medium* demonstrated that there was DNA present in the

Rous tumor agent, characteristic of bacteria. (Alexander-Jackson, 1970) Why was it still being called a virus?

When Livingston confronted Rous that his "retrovirus" could be dried, shelved, stored and mixed months later in saline only to grow out on bacterial culture plates, he reminded her that he had never said it was a virus, carefully using "tumor agent".

To be certain, the Livingston network concluded that oncogenic, supposedly cancer-causing viruses were in fact L-forms of the mycobacteria and related organisms. And they came much too close to proving their point to suit American retrovirologists.

HIV co–discoverer Robert Gallo, threatened, huffed: "What is going on in this country? This is insanity! She can have her theories and what can I say? I don't know of anything to support it. I can't see any basis and I don't know what to say or what analogy to give you." (Parachini, 1984) But Livingston's findings, with worldwide stature, were not about the theory of retroviruses yet to be isolated. She had, in fact, come much closer than any of the retrovirologists in proving a direct causation between her organism and cancer by showing that it manufactured human growth hormone, long associated with malignancy. (Livingston 1974)

Before her death, Livingston would give one more clue towards unraveling what had become AIDS. There were "less known", "little publicized" microorganisms that were transmitted sexually. Through bacteriological studies she had confirmed that the very same L-forms of mycobacteria she found in Rous, by some called mycoplasma, could be found in the semen of man. (Livingston, 1972)

4/ IN THE SEMEN OF MAN

Although tuberculosis was rarely thought of as sexually transmitted, the potential for this had always existed. In the presence of prostatitis, it may be transmitted through the semen. (Lattimer & Colmore, 1954)

Anyone who watched AIDS evolve in not only gay America but heterosexually in Africa and Asia could not help but be struck by its travel and spread along the epidemiologic highways of sex, drugs, migrants, prostitutes, bath houses and venereal disease clinics.

Yet the realization that sexual transmission of AIDS could occur between a man with risk factors and a woman came late. (CDC, 1983) Soon thereafter, female to male transmission, originally thought unlikely, was also found to occur. (Piot & Quinn, 1984) By 1984, the pivotal importance female prostitutes played in the propagation of AIDS in Equatorial Africa had become evident. (Van de Peere & Clumeck, 1985)

But despite the magnifying forces of high tech tests such as The Polymerase Chain Reaction (PCR), which are protein broths which make multiple copies of hard to find pathogens, and which critics contest vastly exaggerates HIV by making numerous copies of fragments of nucleic acid which might or might not even be HIV, HIV can be detected only in a distinct minority of semen samples: one in twenty-five. (Van Voorhis & Martinez, 1991)

On the other hand, ignored and unnoticed, the very real possibility of the genital transmission of *M. tuberculosis*, a disease affecting almost 2 billion people, intimately linked with and considered a reliable sign of AIDS (CDC, 1986; CDC, 1987), and frequently found in the genitourinary tract. (Wyngaarden, 1992) Tuberculosis and *Mycobacterium avium* (also called *Mycobacterium avium-*

intracellulare or MAI and *Mycobacteium avium complex* or MAC) are not only the recognized leading causes of infectious disease in AIDS today; they are by far the most important infections in AIDS.

THE RESEARCH CENTER FOR GENITO-URINARY TUBERCULOSIS
KINGSBRIDGE VETERANS HOSPITAL
BRONX, NEW YORK
1954

By 1954, a pattern emerged at Dr. John Lattimer's Center for Genitourinary Tuberculosis. Men who developed tuberculous epididymitis (inflammation of the testicles) were usually found to have an active focus of tubercular infection in their prostate and cultures of their semen were frequently positive for tubercle bacilli. (Lattimer & Colmore, 1954)

Documenting sexual transmission, what puzzled John Lattimer most was why more husbands with prostatic TB weren't infecting their wives. Two possibilities came to mind. First, the resistance of the thick stratified vaginal epithelium to tubercular infection; second, the scorched earth policy of prostatic tuberculosis, whereby it sought to destroy glandular elements of the prostate (Ibid), severely decreasing semen volume. Many of his male patients, in fact, complained that orgasm produced only slight moisture at the tip of their penis with over half of his experimental groups having a semen volume of less than 0.5cc: too scanty to infect the vaginal or vulvar epithelium, if it reached them at all. As almost a testament to this finding, of 40 men in his practice with tuberculosis genital infections, only one produced a child. (Ibid)

Nevertheless, seeing sexual spread in a disease with staggering numbers right in front of him, he gave notice

Chapter 4/ IN THE SEMEN OF MAN
L. Broxmeyer, M.D.

to the scientific world. (Lattimer & Colmore, 1954) But few listened and adequate descriptions of tuberculosis as a sexually transmitted disease never really reached medical texts.

<u>NIAGARA PENINSULA SANATORIUM</u>
<u>ST. CATHARINES, ONTARIO, CANADA</u>
<u>DECEMBER 1954</u>

Dr. Edgar T. Peer was more than a bit skeptical as he reviewed Lattimer's study regarding the seminal transmission of tuberculosis.

He himself had recovered tubercle bacilli from a patient's semen in 1952, but dismissed the finding as lab error. He would later write that like most dismissals of the tubercle bacilli on similar grounds, it would come back to haunt him.

By 1954, Peer's cases of sexually transmitted tuberculosis were mounting and struck by similarities beyond coincidence, he saw an "extremely probable source" of tuberculosis coming from the male genital tract.

Peer published, warning that if physicians did not wake up to the possibility of sexually transmitted genital tuberculosis, its diagnosis would continue to be unsuspected and underestimated, (Peer, 1957) which one day could lead to potentially catastrophic penalty.

Nor were Peer and Lattimer alone. Netter mentioned that the spread of the tubercle bacilli through the female genital tract of the tubercle bacilli by coitus with a tuberculosis male could not be denied. (Netter, 1987) In fact, wherever culture of the seminal fluid showed *Mycobacterium tuberculosis*, there was a possibility of transmission of genital tuberculosis from male to female

Chapter 4/ IN THE SEMEN OF MAN
L. Broxmeyer, M.D.

via the semen through sexual intercourse. (Chakravarty & Sircar, 1968) While Lattimer (1954) and Peer (1957) showed that the development of tuberculosis ulcers in the vagina or vulva resulting in swollen lymph nodes in the groin were due to semen positive males harboring *M. tuberculosis,* Hellerstrom clocked the actual incubation period from the date of coitus during which the wife was exposed, to the development of vaginal or vulval ulcer and enlargement of inguinal lymph nodes at approximately three to four weeks. (Hellerstrom, 1937)

Heins offered a better idea of the potential potency of sexually transmitted mycobacteria as tuberculosis, demonstrating that even the tame *Mycobacteria smegmatis* found in the smegma genital secretions of both men and women, when introduced into the vaginas of female mice, resulted in the immediate death of over half of an experimental group of 14. (Heins & Dennis, 1958)

Lattimer's cases were compiled from European and American literature. The ulcer and enlarged nodes in the female, often misdiagnosed, closely resembled lymphogranuloma inguinale, syphilis or chancroids, (Ibid) diseases that could coexist with tubercular sexually transmitted disease. (Lattimer & Colmore, 1954)

And, just as men could transmit mycobacterial disease to women, so too could women infect men. (Lewis, 1946) By 1870 Soloweitschnick had documented the first observation of a tuberculosis ulceration of the penis. (Brunati, 1937)

Lewis cited 110 cases of tuberculosis of the penis written up before 1946. Twenty-nine additional cases were subsequently reported by Lal. (Lal & Sekhon, 1971) In his series of primary cases, Lewis pointed to 14 of venereal origin – 12 penile ulcerations being definitely the result of coitus and 2 as a result of oral sex. (Lewis, 1946)

Penile ulcers attributed to primary HIV (Hirschel, 1999) were already well–documented in the TB literature. (Lewis, 1946; Jaisanker,1994; Wood, 1991; Jeyakumar, 1988) And "giant cells" claimed to originate from HIV (Popovic, 1984; Lifson & Reyes, 1986) were decades ago seen at the base of these ulcers. (Lewis, 1946) Long a hallmark of tuberculosis, multi-nucleated giant cells form and engulf the tubercle bacilli in an attempt to kill them. (Livingston, 1972)

Lewis mentions that of all the ways in which the penis could be infected with tubercle bacilli, direct contact was by far the most common.

Although he documented transmission mostly through vaginal and occasionally oral sex, rectal transmission was not explored. (Lewis, 1946)

To explain cases claimed not to arise from direct vaginal inoculation, woman to man, Lewis borrowed from Verneuil's hypothesis, somehow overlooked by later writers. In 1883, Verneuil, in *Hypothesis On the Origin of Genital Tuberculosis In The Two Sexes*, proposed a mechanism whereby men with infected urine or semen first inoculated the vaginal vault of their partners, and then, through subsequent sex became themselves re-inoculated at the corona or frenulum of their own penises. (Verneuil, 1883)

Years passed. Voices of warning persisted.

By 1972, five years before gays started dying in the U.S., Rolland wrote Genital Tuberculosis, a Forgotten Disease? (Rolland, 1972) And ironically, in 1979, on the eve of AIDS recognition, Gondzik and Jasiewicz showed that even in the laboratory, genitally infected tubercular male guinea pigs could infect healthy females through their semen by an HIV-compatible ratio of 1 in 6 or 17%, prompting him to warn his patients that not only was tuberculosis probably a sexually transmitted disease, but also the necessity of the application of suitable contraceptives such as condoms to avoid it. (Gondsik, 1979)

Gondzik's solution and date of publication are chilling; his findings significant. Even in syphilis at its most infectious stage, successful transmission in humans was only possible in 30% of contacts. (Smith, 1988)

Two years later, investigators in South Africa, itself perched on the precipice of a devastating sexually transmitted AIDS epidemic, issued a report of 91 cases of tuberculosis of the penis. (Morrison, 1974; Wilson-Jones, 1986) This was followed by documentation in which "HIV" in young African females came only after first contracting genital TB. (Giannacupoulos, 1998)

Moreover, that *Mycobacterium avium-intracellulare*– fowl or swine tuberculosis, considered an "atypical" tuberculosis could also act like a sexually transmitted disease, set up an explosive scenario. (DePaepe, 1990; De Caprariis, 1984; Damsker, 1985)

Avium had, in the short space of 30 years gone from relative obscurity to the leading infectious disease in U.S. AIDS. And despite the fact that DePaepe's group only used conventional Ziehl-Neelsen stain without culture of either testicular tissue or semen, they still found *M. avium* in these specimens in 32% of AIDS patients with systemic *M. avium,* the same *M. avium* that would eventually kill most U.S. AIDS patients that did not die from one or another AIDS–related disease. (Nightingale, 1992)

Chapter 4/ IN THE SEMEN OF MAN
L. Broxmeyer, M.D.

<u>QUEENS HOSPITAL CENTER</u>
<u>LONG ISLAND JEWISH-HILLSIDE MEDICAL CENTER</u>
<u>JAMAICA, NEW YORK</u>
<u>1984</u>

Dr. Pascal De Caprariis saw before him a dying 30-year-old Haitian man with AIDS. A biopsy of the lymph node in the patient's groin showed *Mycobacterium avium-intracellulare* gone systemic, spreading to the liver. Despite using different combinations totaling 7 different anti-mycobacterials, the patient died.

Then, just before death an ulcerative lesion of the corona of the penis formed. Tests for herpes were negative. Upon culture and only upon culture, *Mycobacteria avium* was isolated from the penile crater, and De Caprariis started speculating that with this and the right groin lymphatic swelling, sexual transmission of *Avium* seemed neither far-fetched nor improbable. (De Caprariis, 1984)

<u>DEPARTMENT OF MICROBIOLOGY</u>
<u>MOUNT SINAI HOSPITAL</u>
<u>NEW YORK</u>
<u>1985</u>

Avium, although ubiquitous, was also in animal reservoirs, swine among them. (Chapman, 1977) For American microbiologist Beca Damsker, who found overwhelming mycobacterial infections of the colon and rectal tissues in U.S. gay AIDS patients time and again, an anorectal portal of transmission had to be considered important. She had, with regularity, found *Avium* or swine tuberculosis in gay stool and biopsy specimens. (Damsker, 1985) There was also the specter of the predilection of some homosexuals for bestiality, sexual activities with animals, a potential vector of transmission to man, which when combined with the fragility of the rectal mucosa to local trauma or intercourse and antigenic challenge (Mavligit & Talpaz, 1984), could bring calamitous unchecked increase of *M. avium-intracellulare*, possibly of animal origin, in the intestinal mucosa, later spreading into the blood with resultant targeting of other systems. (Damsker, 1985)

Tuberculosis in swine is almost always caused by *M. avium* (Karlson, 1968) and such avian tuberculosis leads to some of the highest financial losses in the swine and poultry farm industry. (Berthelsen, 1974)

Although *M. avium-Intracellulare* was thought of as an "opportunistic" infection which occurred only late in the immunosuppression of AIDS, Damsker encouraged a better analysis of the temporal relationship between *M. avium-intracellulare* infection and American AIDS, foreseeing that what doctors were documenting in AIDS could be nothing but a stepwise increment of *Mycobacteria avim-intracellulare*, present from the beginning but ever increasing, both in the scope of its infection, immune suppression, and lowered CD4 count. (Damsker, 1985) In theorizing such, Beca Damsker presented a very possible cause for AIDS.

5/ CATS

In the Europe and the U.S. of the early 1980's, a viral AIDS witch hunt was on, and a few retrovirologists, strategically located at the CDC, National Institute of Health (NIH) and Harvard School of Public Health, joined ranks to force-feed a new option, a retrovirus.

William Jarrett, a veterinarian scientist from the University of Glasgow, reported a "virus-like particle" associated with cat leukemia, (Jarrett, 1964) but also found in many healthy cats.

This particle would come to be called feline leukemic virus (FeLV) or Jarrett virus leukemia and was classified as a retrovirus which at times seemed to provoke malignant change, prevent cell development and cause immune suppression in cats. (Jarrett, 1969; Jarrett, 1970) Most veterinarians did not speculate on the cause of human illness.........for obvious reasons. But this standard was broken when Jarrett and his brother Oswald collaborated with Myron Essex and William Hardy to further study FeLV. Soon veterinarian turned Harvard retroviral researcher Myron "Max" Essex, doing further "cat house" studies, saw what he felt was a parallel between feline leukemic virus and what was happening in human AIDS. He discussed his findings with Dr. Robert Gallo.

Thus the possibility of an AIDS retrovirus was born from a shaky leap in imagination that what Essex and Jarrett had found earlier in cats was now happening in humans.

In the background, Jane Teas, another researcher, like Essex, from the Harvard School of Public Health, deduced that AIDS was due to the African Swine Flu Virus (ASFV). (Teas, 1983) Teas however, would be quickly drowned out by the retroviral cat fanciers.

Chapter 5/ CATS
L. Broxmeyer, M.D.

The holes in the cat retroviral theory were enormous. Not only was it commonly found in normal healthy cats (Duesberg, 1987), but in one report "feline leukemic virus" (FeLV) could be nursed out of two-thirds of cancerous cats, one-third being virus negative. (Francis, 1979) Why one-third of the malignant cats had no virus was unclear to everyone except the retroviral researchers who were certain that the cancer was still being caused by FeLV. Moreover, it has been estimated that at least 50-60% of cats, or more at some point, became naturally infected by Feline Leukemic Virus (Rogerson, 1975), yet only approximately 0.4% of all cats developed leukemia annually in their short lives. (Dorn, 1968)

Although these animal scientists spoke of AIDS caused from "an infectious agent, presumably a virus", their continued bombardment of the media about a feline leukemia/lymphoma virus which few medical doctors understood, spoke with more certainty than presumption and as Essex and his cat experiments faded, National Cancer Institute (NCI) retrovirologist Robert Gallo took up the banner in the form of his leukemic/lymphomic human retroviruses, HTLV1 and HTLV2.

Few realized that latent retroviruses were the most common nonpathogenic passenger viruses of either healthy animals or humans and were frequent harmless passenger viruses in not only AIDS, but cat, cow and human leukemias as well. (Duesberg, 1987)

Even before Koch discovered the causative organism of human tuberculosis in 1882, it was recognized in dogs and cats. (Blaine, 1913) Up to 13% of cats (Snider, 1971) harbored the disease, often unsuspected. In most it spread to the lymph nodes but it could also enter the cats genital tract in which case it assumed the capacity to become a sexually transmitted disease. (Robin, 1954)

Often, a rapid course of cat death occurred, 10 to 20 days from the onset of symptoms. (Snider, 1971)

Recognized by Jordan (1994), cat tubercular and mycobacterial infection had, like all mycobacteria, retroviral-like L forms, could immunosuppress (Drolet, 1986) simulate cancer (Miller, 1999), and had its own opportunistic disease.

It soon became obvious that cats were also susceptible to *Avium* tuberculosis, a leading cause of infection and death in American AIDS. (Hix, 1961) (Jordan, 1994) (Malik, 1998)

By 1978, just prior to the recognition of the AIDS epidemic, Robert Gallo, isolating a human retrovirus from T cell Leukemia in the blood of a cancer patient, named it HTLV1. Problem was, it didn't cause the leukemia (Sezary T-cell Leukemia) from which it was isolated, only appearing in a small fraction of cases, and was found in many, many healthy people.

HTLV1 was now a retrovirus without a disease. But soon, Gallo and colleagues, Essex among them, would suggest it as the probable cause of AIDS. Never mind that its prevalence in AIDS was no more than 25% and that just finding antibodies for it in AIDS blood was hit–and–miss.

As it turned out HTLV1, despite its growing literature, did not cause AIDS, and the main fear of these AIDS retrovirologists at this point was that their retrovirus would prove to be just another "opportunistic" infection lurking behind the real cause of AIDS, something the CDC was already preparing to report. (CDC, 1983) In fact, Walter Dowdle, then Chief of CDC, thought that his center had put too much time and emphasis into the retroviral hypothesis altogether.

Chapter 5/ CATS
L. Broxmeyer, M.D.

That same year French scientists, racing back from a New York AIDS Symposium that spoke of a causal human leukemic retrovirus (HTLV) decided to enlist the help of retrovirologists at the famed Pasteur Institute. Pointing out the one true direction to go after a disease that destroyed the T-4 helper lymphocytes in the blood was the lymph nodes themselves, they pursued Luc Montagnier, Head of Cancer Virology.

6/ TRAGIC COST OF PREMATURE CONSENSUS

<u>PASTEUR INSTITUTE</u>
<u>PARIS</u>
<u>JANUARY, 1983</u>

The Pasteur Institute squeezed head of cancer virology Luc Montagnier into the pressure cooker of finding an AIDS retrovirus after its production of Hepatitis B vaccine, accounting for a significant part of its income, in part processed from pooled American homosexual blood, came under fire.

Montagnier, unsuspectingly looking for a virus closely related to Gallo's HTLV-1, instead came upon LAV (Lymphadenopathy Associated Virus), first identified by Francoise Barre-Sinoussi, a member of his team at Pasteur's Virology.

LAV was so named because the French homosexual fashion designer it was first isolated from had enlarged, inflamed neck nodes (lymphadenopathy), a common, early, AIDS feature. Thirty-three and promiscuous, he had also visited New York City in 1979 and had a 50-gay-partner-a-year history.

Betting the obvious, that the agent responsible for AIDS could be more readily detected in these swollen lymph nodes, Barre, in January, 1983, packed a small piece of the homosexual's just biopsied lymph node *en Toto* in ice at Paris's Pitie-Salpetriere Hospital and delivered it to Montagnier at Pasteur. This patient did not yet have full-blown AIDS, but his history and symptoms were strongly suggestive. (Barre-Sinoussi, 1983) He would die 5 years later of the disease.

At Pasteur, Montagnier put the tissue into cell cultures of T-lymphocytes. Immediately questions arose as to procedure. Looking only for a retrovirus, the team cultured whole tissue lymph node lysates. The "virus" was never isolated in its pure form. It would be the beginning of a long, long line of research work based on indirect evidence.

Later, looking at Montagnier's tissue cultures microscopically there were many granules, some of which were felt to look like retroviruses; but they were inside cells and tissues – not whole viral particles and had different shapes and sizes. No two were alike. They seemed to show all forms of "viral maturation", but were they viral?

As early as 1928, Eleanor Alexander-Jackson began discovering unusual, and to that point, unrecognized forms of the TB Bacillus. Jackson marveled at the many forms of tuberculosis, including the tiny granules which the German Much saw in 1908 and soon became known as Much's granules. (Much, 1931) In 1910 Fontes proved Much's granules, as a sub-classification of Kleinberger's L-forms were filterable and therefore also often mistaken for viruses. In fact, in certain circles the variable acid-fast granules were called 'the TB virus'. (Fontes, 1910)

Even prior to Livingston (1970), Mellon and Fisher had warned that filterable forms of *M. avium* and *M. tuberculosis* could easily be mistaken for the virus Montagnier and Barre thought they had, (Mellon and Fisher, 1932) and might explain "the common finding by French workers of acid-fast bacilli in the glands of guinea-pigs into which viral-like, cell-free filtrates of tuberculosis material had been injected". (Ibid)

7/ THE RACE

The race was on. Gallo's leukemic retrovirus (HTLV), which Barre and Montagnier thought they had isolated, should have led to the wild proliferation of lymphocytes. But all that Barre found in subsequent trips to the lab was how well it was slaughtering them. What also puzzled her was that retroviruses typically didn't kill cells. How could she explain this?

By January 25th, 1983, Barre's reverse transcriptase radioactivity counter was showing increased numbers, to her meaning the "retrovirus" LAV was multiplying.

But reverse transcriptase was nonspecific and was also found elevated in events leading to the death of CD4 lymphocytes by tuberculosis (Watson, 2000), as well as in *M. avium* infection of neck lymph nodes (April, 1996), probably the very event Barre was watching. Why had she not considered these as possible AIDS causes?

In actuality, previously having been viral cancer researchers, Barre and Montagnier were solely attuned, intellectually and technologically to detecting retroviruses. Barre had been trained in mouse retroviral techniques requiring the measurement of reverse transcriptase in Robert Bassin's National Cancer Institute (NCI) lab. Her procedures were not designed to explore for some unknown pathogen. In effect, Barre and Montagnier found a retrovirus because that was all that they were looking for.

Within weeks Montagnier called a staff meeting. The new "retrovirus" wasn't Gallo's HTLV. He didn't assert that his group had proved that LAV caused AIDS, but it was possible. In the future he would send samples of the tissue culture to Gallo who headed AIDS research at NCI to stimulate further research.

Approximately one year later, after receiving French samples from Montagnier, retrovirologist Gallo isolated and announced HTLV-3 as the AIDS retrovirus, which proved to be the same as LAV: a productive Lentivirus infection with all forms of viral maturation.

A colleague suggested that Montagnier characterize his virus as a Lentivirus (Lenti means slow) on a hunch. Lentiviruses were large viruses that, after entering cells, did not leap into activity at once, but later shot into action.

But so-called slow viruses had been implicated, but never proven, in diseases such as Creutzfeldt-Jacob and Alzheimer's. Prominent American retrovirologist Peter Duesberg, who did much of the pioneer work on retroviral ultrastructure, knew that retroviruses were not "slow" viruses, even lentiviruses like visna with which HIV was often compared. Rather, if Visna reached high enough blood concentration, it was rapidly pathogenic. (Lairmore, 1986) HIV, however, was not to be found in such high blood titer. Perplexed, Duesberg summed that there was no such thing as a slow virus, "only slow virologists". (Health Education AIDS Liaison, 2001)

The discovery of LAV (HIV) allowed virologists to take the high ground in American medicine. No longer would practicing physicians like Livingston, who had seen disease face to face, assume leadership on policy issues. The new medical shamans would be laboratory gene splicers, molecular biologists, virologists and immunologists who told doctors what to think. A dangerous precedent was being set.

Chapter 7/ THE RACE
L. Broxmeyer, M.D.

Former viral cancer researcher Abraham Karpas, worked out of the Department of Hematological Medicine at Cambridge. By September 1983 he had identified a "transmissible agent" through electron micrographs of the blood of a gay AIDS patient. (Karpas, 1983)

Karpas was having a problem with Gallo's HTLV1 and was unable to confirm previous reports of this purported AIDS retrovirus in Africans. Many blood tests finding HTLV1 positive by previous investigators where found negative when retested in Karpas's lab. (Karpas, 1986)

Karpas, probably the second man in the world to see the AIDS agent, fired off a quick report on hIs transmissible agent complete with a microphotograph, but was having difficulty getting the paper published. He had the honesty to admit that he wasn't certain that the 55nm particles with their 10nm electrodense cores were viruses at all and began his paper with the phrase "assuming it is a virus," though he later found them identical to Montagnier's HIV.

Experts sided with Karpas's restraint. Not only were retroviral particles not proof that such particles were viral but such particles were ubiquitous – a statement supported by O'Hara's Harvard study which found "viral particles, morphologically indistinguishable" in 90% of the enlarged lymph nodes in both AIDS and non-AIDS patients. (O'Hara, 1988)

O'Hara's study stood out as the one study to date which used suitable controls, finding 'viral particles' indistinguishable from HIV in a variety of swollen lymph nodes without HIV.

Similarly, African studies of the lymph nodes of patients with HIV also showed viral particles indistinguishable from those with just tuberculosis and without AIDS. (Nambuya, 1988; Voetberg, 1991) O'Hara concluded, "The presence of such particles do not, by themselves, indicate infection with HIV." Yet it was micrographs of these same particles which first informed the world that there was an HIV.

In <u>Reproduction of RNA Tumor Viruses</u>, Badar warned that *in vitro* cultures, even virus free, "can be induced to produce particles which resemble RNA tumor viruses in every physical and chemical respect", (Bader, 1975) an event many saw applicable to the rigors Montagnier and Gallo put their AIDS tissues thru.

Oddly, It was not until 1997 that two independent groups examined these HIV particles in accordance with accepted international procedure. (Gluschankof, 1997; Bess, 1997) Both teams saw an excess of fluid filled, many formed (pleomorphic) 'contaminating' vesicles, ranging in size from 50 to 500 nm as opposed to a minor population of particles of about 100nm.

The latter were assumed to be viral, but proved, according to critics, to be too large, the wrong shape and containing too much material to be retroviruses. In fact, both the particles and vesicles of Bess and Gluschankof shared common antigenic determinants and could easily have been, and do seem reminiscent of the variably acid-fast mycobacterial L-forms pointed out and electronically microphotographed by Seibert (1970), Alexander-Jackson (1954), Livingston (1972) and Cantwell (1981). Livingston showed a protoplast with L-form inclusions budding out vesicles from its surface not unlike the vesicles in the 1997 AIDS verification studies, while Seibert and Cantwell showed particles similar to those attributed to

HIV. And the 'substantial amount' of both RNA and DNA found by Bess points to bacterial or mycobacterial origin.

Suddenly, it seemed as if the world had been sold a bill of sale on a non-existent virus.

8/ INVISIBLE VIRUS

By 1984, one year before some of America's finest scientists split from the retroviral theory of AIDS, HIV scientists faced an embarrassment of substantial proportions. It had become evident that Kaposi's Sarcoma (KS) cells were not infected with HIV.

After all, a key reason the retroviral theory of AIDS was brought forward to begin with was that HIV was claimed to be the sole cause of early opportunistic infections, particularly *Pneumocystis* and Kaposi's Sarcoma (KS) in previously healthy persons. (CDC, 1982) Kaposi's at one time attacked up to one-third of all AIDS patients.

Now felt to be a specific sexually transmitted agent other than HIV (Beral, 1990), KS is attributed to an unknown infectious agent.

This conclusion was reached only after it became obvious that the AIDS clinical syndrome, including specific, frequent conditions such as Kaposi's and *Pneumocystis Carinii* pneumonia, appeared in HIV negative patients. (Moore & Ho, 1992) But If HIV didn't cause KS, the most frequent cancer in AIDS, then what did? Evidence soon pointed again to the acid-fast mycobacteria.

On autopsy, Cantwell repeatedly found variably acid-fast *Mycobacterium avium* not only in Kaposi's but in a clinically probable case of a never–diagnosed *Pneumocystis carinii* pneumonia or PCP (Cantwell, 1986) *Pneumocystis* was never isolated from the lungs of his deceased 36–year–old patient, but variably acid-fast *M. avium* were. The study, a microcosm of AIDS as it originated in the United States, suggested that acid-fast bacteria might play a role in both the development of Kaposi's Sarcoma (KS) and the inflammatory lung disease *Pneumocystis,* which frequently occurred in homosexual men who died of AIDS.

Chapter 8/ INVISIBLE VIRUS
L. Broxmeyer, M.D.

As a dermatologist/researcher, this was not the first time Cantwell found acid-fast bacteria in Kaposi's.

In 1981, the same year that the AIDS epidemic began, he published two similar studies showing variably acid-fast forms in non-AIDS Kaposi's. (Cantwell, 1981a; Cantwell, 1981b)

Then turning his attention towards Kaposi's in gay men, he found the same organisms. (Cantwell, 1983) A 31-year-old gay man hospitalized at UCLA with fatal AIDS and Kaposi's proved to grow out *Mycobacterium avium* and *Mycobacterium gordonae*: two non-tuberculosis ('atypical') mycobacteria. The case was reported along with seven other autopsied cases of AIDS patients who died at UCLA, all but one showed acid-fast mycobacteria at autopsy. (Zakowski, 1982)

By 1983, Croxson was finding mycobacteria in the spindle-shaped configuration of AIDS Kaposi's. (Croxson, 1983) Croxson concluded that they seemed more causative than opportunistic. This turned out to be the same combination of *M. avium* and *M. gordonae* previously seen in Cantwell's UCLA patient.

The coordinated attack of two mycobacteria on the same victim, ever more familiar, was again being documented. (Tsukamura, 1981)

And the fact that dapsone, a first line drug for acid–fast *Mycobacteria Leprae* (Leprosy) was curing Kaposi's in AIDS was further proof that Kaposi's was a mycobacterial disease (*The Lancet*: March 10, 1984)

Chen and Shieh found these same mycobacteria in fatal Kaposi's in an HIV negative patient who had rapidly ulcerating anal papules. (Chen, 2000) Evidence was beginning to mount and it wasn't just in Kaposi's.

Chapter 8/ INVISIBLE VIRUS
L. Broxmeyer, M.D.

By 1982 Cantwell found acid-fast forms in the enlarged neck nodes of a young male homosexual first diagnosed with the ever–present 'reactive lymph node hyperplasia': the inflamed lymph nodes so prevalent in early gay AIDS. (Cantwell, 1982)

Subsequently, Cantwell again isolated mycobacterial-like forms throughout the tissues of a 48-year-old AIDS homosexual whose body had been teeming with them. (Cantwell, 1983)

Concurrently, Cohen, in San Francisco, mapped 7 AIDS patients whose bone marrows were imbedded with *Avium*, speaking of the difficulties of finding this organism without proper acid-fast stains. (Cohen, 1983) At the same time Cohen recommended acid-fast staining for every AIDS patient that had a bone marrow biopsy.

It seemed that everywhere AIDS went, mycobacteria followed; or were they causing it?

9/ SMOKE AND MIRRORS

Like chameleons, HIV scientists continued to change their colors to blend into whatever new facts came along, much of it from the mycobacterial literature found in AIDS. And since the doctors and scientists who bought into the HIV theory were in the clear majority, and that majority ruled, their funding and literature mushroomed, not unlike that of the already disproven HTLV1, into a self-fulfilling archive while those that did not agree found themselves labeled heretics, lost tenure, research funding and even their jobs.

By 1983, the certain knowledge that AIDS had begun its wholesale slaughter of Africans mainly through heterosexual sex sent shudders down the back of a world in which, not since the last great sexual pandemic of syphilis five centuries ago, had there been anything comparable.

Men and woman were transmitting AIDS back and forth sexually in heretofore-unheralded numbers.

Wave after wave of epidemic tuberculosis had hit the world. It was a disease of big numbers. In the 100 years from 1850-1950, an estimated 1 billion persons died from tuberculosis. (Iseman, 1994)

From England it spread to the shores of Western and then Eastern Europe and by 1900, North and South American waves began to peak. But in the developing countries of Asia and Africa, where the AIDS epidemic was new in 1983, epidemic waves of tuberculosis had not yet reached their zenith. (Stead, 1983) As this epidemic continued to seethe, it was these very countries that would show the highest TB mortality and morbidity, even before AIDS came into the picture (Lowell, 1976), and would prove to be the future epicenters for AIDS.

Foreigners called the all-too-common African AIDS wasting syndrome "slim disease"; Africans just "slim". Serwadda wrote about it in <u>Slim Disease: a New Disease in Uganda</u> (Serwadda, 1985) but of 82 patients diagnosed with this wasting syndrome, he found 44% to have disseminated tuberculosis. Referring to what he felt to be the tip of an iceberg, Serwadda suggested that a substantial proportion, if not all, Slim Disease was due to disseminated tuberculosis. (DeCock, 1992) In addition, disseminated *M. Avium* too was believed to be a major cause of wasting syndrome in patients with AIDS with approximately 40% having nausea or diarrhea. (Kemper, 1992; Modilevsky, 1989)

True, tuberculosis and diarrhea, prominent in African AIDS, had been killing African's for some time, but suddenly African TB had become untreatable. A new name was needed for an old affliction. And that name, AIDS, was supplied, hurriedly, perhaps too hurriedly.

It was in Africa that those who hailed HIV as the cause of AIDS faced their first and most serious challenge over extremely suspicious coincidences. Not only were over 65% of African AIDS patients not HIV-positive, (*Lancet*, Oct. 17, 1992) but, of those that tested positive, data suggested that the antigens in HIV-1 Elisa and Western Blots, initially claimed to belong solely to HIV, were in fact cross-reacting with the mycobacteria. (Kashala, 1994)

Mycobacterial cell wall components, phenolic glycolipid (PGL) and lipoara-binomannan (LAM) were noted not only to strongly cross-react with p24, the sacred cow of 'HIV isolation', but p31, also favored in the detection of HIV in the blood. (Kashala, 1994)

Chapter 9/ SMOKE AND MIRRORS
L. Broxmeyer, M.D.

Even the most prominent and persistently detected antigen in AIDS tests (Veronese, 1985) p41, could be found in bacteria such as tuberculosis.

Defensively, HIV enthusiasts shot back that tuberculosis in AIDS was merely an "opportunistic infection", a label that most North American AIDS experts were originally extremely reluctant to assign. To John and Kaur, in a *Lancet* article, the term "opportunistic" seemed inappropriate. Infections due to non-disease-causing microbes were "opportunistic". (John, 1993)

Mycobacterium tuberculosis was the only infectious pathogen ever to force the UN to issue a (1993) global emergency.

Many physicians, wary of the invented terms used to describe HIV, still remained silent.

Makeshift expressions, like ARC (Aids Related Complex), and "pre-AIDS" were scrutinized in disbelief. There were similar forms of latent TB, yet none were ready to call them pre-tuberculosis or TRC (Tuberculosis–Related Complex).

By 1986 Montagnier's group, puzzled, found a patient in West Africa with AIDS but no HIV antibodies in the blood. Rather than rethink the whole HIV hypothesis, the discoverer of HIV proceeded to simply say that it was another retrovirus at work: HIV2, said to be responsible for a large West African epidemic, mainly transmitted through heterosexual intercourse. (Clavel, 1986)

Lacor Hospital in Gulu, Uganda was in effect a TB sanitarium, but roughly half of the patients who remained there for two months or more came down with AIDS. And so Africans died, with the bleeding gums and anemia claimed at different times to come from both HIV and TB, but their blood was HIV–negative. In a word, they died of wasting..........or consumption.

———————————————————

10/ AMBIGUOUS SLAUGHTER

The scientific vagueness and deception to bolster the HIV theory continued.

Important to the basic mechanism of AIDS is the destruction of CD4 (T-cell) lymphocytes, key to the body's resistance against infection. As this CD4 cell count falls in the blood of an AIDS patient, many treacherous infections are able to jump on board.

HIV was early on claimed to destroy these CD4 white blood cells, yet the exact mechanism for this was never made clear. (Jaworowski, 1999)

What Papadopulos-Eleopulos makes clear is that retroviruses were never known to kill cells. It was the one thing retrovirologists always knew and agreed upon. Therefore, she asked, how could they kill CD4? Instead, it seemed to her that CD4 T–Lymphocyte death might be due to the many non-HIV factors present in HIV inoculate, including other infectious agents. (Papadopulos-Eleopulus, 1995)

And although low CD4 has been made synonymous with HIV by many, the fact is that known AIDS-risk groups may have low CD4 even in the face of persistently negative HIV antibody tests. (Detels, 1988; Donahoe, 1987; Novick, 1986)

That HIV is not the cause of apoptosis (or immune cell destruction) of CD4+ is indicated by the fact that in chronically infected retroviral cell lines, where HIV is continually produced, apoptosis is not to be detected. (Papadopulos-Eleopulos, 1995)

Discoverer Luc Montagnier and others have confirmed that HIV does not kill T-cells like CD4+ directly. (Lemaitre et al., 1990; Duesberg, 1992)

Chapter 10/ AMBIGUOUS SLAUGHTER
L. Broxmeyer, M.D.

On the other hand, virulent TB can depress the CD4 count, (WHO, 1989) and does kill T-cells like CD4+ directly, as well as macrophages through nitric oxide secretion. (Rojas, 1999)

In 1978, the first European measurement of a low CD4 in AIDS was on a patient with disseminated atypical *Mycobacteria fortuitum* (Bultmann, 1982), closely related to *Mycobacterium tuberculosis.*

By 1987, researchers realized that mycobacteria such as tuberculosis alone could be responsible for direct CD4 killing and much of the immunosuppression found in AIDS. Furthermore, such a tubercular immune system throttle could persist for life, even when the disease wasn't progressive. (Lamoureux, 1987)

In the same vein, Mudaki, in Zaire, showed how fast a CD4 count could shrink below 200/ul just by tuberculosis, without HIV. (Mudaki, 1993) Moreover, TB often presented before the development of immune dysfunction, either with or without HIV. (Reeve, 1993)

In fact of all the infections involved in AIDS, none were associated with as low CD4 cell counts as were mycobacterial infections. (Ohtomo, 2000) And those patients with either *M. avium* or *M. tuberculosis* in their blood had significantly lower CD4 counts. (Gilks, 1995)

Yet there had to be more – a missing link. It has long been known that a low CD4 count in and of itself did not by itself lead to the severe immunodepression found in AIDS. (John, 1993)

CASE WESTERN RESERVE UNIVERISITY
OHIO
JULY, 1998

Chapter 10/ AMBIGUOUS SLAUGHTER
L. Broxmeyer, M.D.

Although previously demonstrated (Lamoureux, 1987; Dlugovitsky, 1995), the ferocity of a tubercular attack shown in papers such as Hirsh's 1999 Ohio study amplified that not only were 30% of CD4 and non–CD4 cells slaughtered within 98 hours of co-culture with TB, a 20–fold increase, (Hirsh, 1999) but B cells (McDonald, 1996; Chaouchi, 1995) and macrophages (Molloy, 1994; Fratazzi, 1999) were also decimated.

The fact that both TB specific and non-specific T cells were equally affected would account for tuberculosis's silent role in the depressed responsiveness towards non-TB antigens such as Candidal thrush, *Pnuemocystis*, and other opportunistic organisms; non-CD4 lymphocytes hold a possible role in keeping these at bay.

But it was in the annihilation of infection swallowing macrophages, critical to reticuloendothelial ultra-structure, that *M. tuberculosis*, *M. avium* (Bermudez, 1999), or both working together, furnished the key to AIDS devastation.

CALIFORNIA PACIFIC MEDICAL CENTER RESEARCH INSTITUTE
SAN FRANCISCO, CALIFORNIA
1999

A stagnant HIV hypothesis, much in need of rejuvenation, was expanded to include infection of macrophages, long the home base of tuberculosis and now claimed to be the most important reservoir of the AIDS 'virus' from which a sustained, long term attack on the body's lymphocytes could proceed. (Ho, 1986) Although Duesberg and Levy saw HIV infection of macrophages as possible, their subsequent killing by HIV was not. (Duesberg, 1991; Levy, 1988)

Chapter 10/ AMBIGUOUS SLAUGHTER
L. Broxmeyer, M.D.

Indeed, the missing link in AIDS was the macrophage. It had long been known that certain white blood cells called macrophages ate (phagocytosed) bacteria. But how tuberculosis and the mycobacteria, naturally endowed with their own thick, lipid–rich cell envelopes, became mankinds greatest assassins ever, presently responsible for a human death every 15 seconds (www.stoptb.org) relied on how they resisted lysosomal degradation inside the macrophage, multiplied there (Armstrong, 1971), and ate it up, from the inside out. (Gangadharam, 1983) Inside every macrophage swim two thin-membraned vacuoles: one, the phagosome, containing ingested bacteria; the other the lysosome containing lysozyme, a destructive enzyme tailored to kill bacteria. Usually, with infection, the two vacuoles fuse or join, the acidic and enzymatic content of the lysosome killing bacterial elements harbored in the phagosome. It is how the macrophage defends the body. But after eons of evolution virulent mycobacteria and tuberculosis have developed a survival strategy which includes coating the phagosomes they find themselves in with proteins to prevent their enzymatic destruction (Pieters, 2001), punching holes into the phagosomal membrane for nutrition and release of toxic products (Teitelbaum, 1999), evading enzymatic destruction even in those cases where vacular fusion has taken place (Armstrong, 1975), and learning to escape from such fused vacuoles (McDonough, 1933), only to eventually kill the macrophage as the hunter becomes the hunted. Thus TB and the mycobacteria enjoy and thrive in a macrophagal lifestyle deadly to most other pathogens. (Rhoades, 2000)

At California Pacific Research Institute, for example, Bermudez, Parker and Petrofsky slatched ferocious AIDS *Mycobacterium avium* destroy 28 to 46% more macrophages than uninfected cultures. (Bermudez, 1999) And although it was known that both *Avium* and tuberculosis could escape dying macrophages only to kill

          AIDS: WHAT THE DISCOVERERS
OF HIV NEVER ADMITTED

and infect others, in the case of AIDS *Avium,* Bermudez saw a particularly menacing event in front of him: macrophage kill only made *Avium* more virulent and hungrier than ever (Bermudez, 1997) as it sought out its next macrophage victim.

11/ VIRAL MIRAGE

By 1995, David Ho, head of the New York's Aaron Diamond AIDS Research Center, assumed the mantel of titular head of the US AIDS establishment; he and his colleagues proclaiming a new proactive stance, asserting that HIV was never inactive and multiplied astronomically in the body each day, killing CD4 cells. But there was still no hard physical evidence, only theory, as to how HIV killed. Ho speculated that the carnage took place in the lymph nodes, so that there were few signs of infected CD4 in the blood. Then HIV not involved in this hypothesized slaughter shot out into the blood stream, creating a "viral load". To eradicate viral load, Ho was suggesting early and aggressive anti-viral drugs taken in potent "cocktails," with serious side effects, and probably for the life of the patient. The problem was, as Robert Gallo later noted, that just about everyone he knew realized from the start that Ho's theory was absolutely wrong.

Nevertheless, soon HIV scientists were proclaiming that the amount of virus in the blood was the most important determinant in AIDS prognosis. (Lyles, 1999) But the fact is that HIV is so sparse in the blood as to require Polymerase Chain Reaction (PCR), a nucleic acid broth that makes copious copies of hard-to-find pathogens, to even detect it.

PCR inventor Kary Mullis would not support the use of his test to amplify and exaggerate what is being perceived as HIV in measuring "the viral load," as is currently being done. To many, the massive amounts of RNA supposedly representing HIV in the circulation were suspect. Furthermore, dissidents wanted to know if you made a thousand copies of a dollar bill, how many real dollar bills did you still really have?

Chapter 11/ VIRAL MIRAGE
L. Broxmeyer, M.D.

The "viral load test," presently in use only makes copies of fragments of nucleic acids attributed to HIV (Johnson, 1996) does not count HIV itself. Since it does not count HIV itself and other infections, in particular the mycobacteria, can also yield similar nucleic acid fragments, a positive viral load test cannot be regarded as signaling HIV itself. Meanwhile, nobody ever questioned the validity of using a non-quantitative PCR in the detection of another hard to find pathogen............ tuberculosis.

By 1994, British researcher John Kay walked up to a New Hampshire podium before the Proteolytic Enzyme Conference and announced that Hoffman-LaRoche's protease inhibitor RO31-8959, now called saquinavir or Inverase hadn't worked out clinically in an 18-month trial with 400 AIDS patients. (Conlan, 1998) The reason given was that after an initial improvement in symptoms, HIV developed resistance to the agent and that for the time being Roche was imposing a blackout on the disappointing trial. Biochemist Dr. David Rasnick, an expert on the proteases saw things differently. The inhibitors were performing their job as designed and that was to block HIV production. It wasn't mutation or resistance that were the problems, it was that HIV didn't cause AIDS. (Ibid)

By 1984, Rasnick, with extensive protease experience, was in a pivotal position to capitalize on their momentum but quickly decided that to kill a harmless retrovirus was an exercise in futility; often at the risk of severe and as-yet-unknown side-effects, some fatal in animals.

Although it was generally acknowledged by the HIV establishment that by the 1990's Highly Active Antiretroviral Therapy (HAART) made headway in braking the steep rise in both AIDS and AIDS-related deaths in the U.S., no randomized study has ever been done comparing those on these drugs to those that are not. (Regush, 2001) Furthermore, the precipitous drop in AIDS deaths in 1995 predates the introduction of the protease inhibitors, which first came onto the market in late 1996, by one year. This seems much akin to tuberculosis, which began to decrease before any specific measures or drugs were used against it. (Dubos, 1952)

HAART, to be sure, from its onset was palliative. Nevertheless, with HAART, in many cases, the CD4+ count is partially restored and supposedly therefore the necessity for continuing drugs specifically against *M. Avium* in certain cases stopped. But *M. avium* infection rebounds when these anti–HIV drugs are stopped or fail. (Kaplan, 2000) Furthermore, the antiretrovirals in HAART weren't the only agents that could restore a CD4 count. This restoration also occurred in patients with HIV and TB when anti-TB treatment was used, as in John's study where a CD4 count of 89/ul climbed to 760/ul. (John, 1993)

In truth, the entire story has not been nearly unraveled regarding America's potent anti-retroviral drugs. Regush mentions that the antiviral drugs used in cocktails "have antimicrobial properties that could, to varying degrees, target other infections that are common to AIDS". (Regush, 2001)

FDA approval for any of these agents did not require information as to whether they were bacteriocidal. Therefore, studies which show that widespread HAART reduces the risk for TB or may bring about the further decline of TB among persons infected with HIV (Jones, 2000) can never answer with certainty that the reason for this is not some heretofore unknown direct antimycobacterial activity on the part of HAART.

Chapter 11/ VIRAL MIRAGE
L. Broxmeyer, M.D.

For example, in 1999 Bermudez, Parker and Petrofsky documented that the intense macrophage and lymphocyte killing by American AIDS *M. avium* was significantly reduced by protease inhibitors called caspases. (Bermudez, 1999)

These investigators, in effect, established that certain protease inhibitors, a first line of defense against 'HIV' found in HAART were able to curtail *Mycobacteria avium-intracellulare*'s virulence, thus pinpointing a much more specific and satisfying reason as to why, all of a sudden, MAI prophylaxis was not necessary and symptomatic improvement noted then that HAART was "bolstering the immune system". But the question remained: At what price?

———————————

12/ LUCKY

Once upon a time, a small group of politically powerful scientists rammed a flawed theory on the origin and cause of AIDS down America's and then the world's throat.

Yet we are still led to believe that we are fortunate that retroviruses, only discovered in the 1970's, were uncovered just in time to label them the culprit in a killer AIDS epidemic.........lucky that two "HIV's" were discovered in rapid succession and the technology and theory to link AIDS to the HIV retrovirus were fully in place, for the first time in history, only a few years prior to the recognition of the AIDS epidemic.

Lucky? As the 20th anniversary of the first reported AIDS cases passes, AIDS has infected nearly 60 million people of which almost 22 million, including nearly half-a-million Americans have died, and 8,500 AIDS deaths occur daily. Yet the prospects for a cure or vaccine are as remote as they were two decades ago. And although it is currently difficult to find anyone who openly questions HIV as the cause of AIDS, a fast growing number express their doubts privately.

Historically, not that long ago, and at the end of the 19th century, after 150 years of denial, the medical establishment recognized that there were bacteria, and suddenly every disease seemed to be caused by a bacteria. But with the electron microscope, unknown disease was more and more attributed to a virus, often to no avail. Thus it was that scientists were certain that a virus was behind Lyme's disease, Mycoplasma pneumonia, and Legionnaires' disease before their respective bacteria were found.

Chapter 12/ LUCKY
L. Broxmeyer, M.D.

By 1931, Rudenberg, hoping to visualize the polio virus, filed a patent for his electron microscope and during WWII investigators never gave up on an electron search for a cancer virus, despite one dismal failure after another.

Then an AIDS "virus" was found, primarily because it was looked for; and not because it caused AIDS-bolstered by the half-truths, flawed theory and downright hocus-pocus.

HIV scientists cited that "unassailable epidemiological evidence" (Blattner, 1988) has established HIV or a virus as the cause of AIDS, including those epidemiological studies carried out by the CDC on filtered factor VIII blood transfusions for hemophiliacs. Blattner cites Peterman in his article when he said "it is also noteworthy that HIV infection, and not infection with any other infectious agent, is linked to blood transfusion-associated AIDS". (Peterman, 1988) But blood transfusions do not distinguish between HIV and other filterable infectious agents especially, as in the case of mycobacteria, if these other infectious agents are not screened for. Yet, one of the original factor VIII transfusion cases happened in Canton, Ohio, diagnosed as oral thrush and *Mycobacterium avium*. (Elliot, 1983)

John Lattimer could not foresee the unusual situation which decades later, might be involved with the direct insemination of particularly virulent mycobacteria rectally onto the vulnerable one layered epithelium of the prostate during gay sex, nor the hypervirulent strains of AIDS *Mycobacterium tuberculosis* and *Myco*bacterium *avium* that would one day, decades later, be shared in much greater numbers, heterosexually, and in a worldwide epidemic called AIDS. But who could have?

Nor could Gondzik realize the profound significance of warning his patients, on the eve of an AIDS epidemic in

1979 to wear condoms lest they acquire sexually transmitted tuberculosis.

Mycobacterial infections are the main cause of bacterial infection during AIDS (Perronne, 1995); and often precede other infections by 1 to 10 months. (Bishburg, 1986) The fact that two decades after AIDS started killing people, mycobacteria, despite their prevalence in AIDS, are not considered its cause, is in no small part due to the lack of scientists and the lay public to understand the ability of mycobacterial and tubercular infection, once contracted, to lie seemingly dormant for extended lengths of time in humans, (Youmans, 1979) and at the same time begin to melt the immune system. (Lamoureux, 1987)

Nor was it emphasized that both tuberculosis, with chronic lymphadenitis among its most frequent manifistations (Jawahar, 2000), and *M. avium,* the most common cause of lymphadenitis in children (Hazra, 1999) can attack lymph nodes (Terrones, 1997) and the entire body additively and simultaneously. (Tsukamura, 1981)

AIDS is a mycobacterial disease and patients with advanced TB or *Avium* are indistinguishable from those with "HIV". Even in the earliest AIDS cases on record, dating back to 1959, tuberculosis (Williams, 1987) and the atypical mycobacteria (Schoenell, 1968) (Hagmar, 1969) were clinically and bacteriologically diagnosed.

Perhaps one of the most convincing arguments for the intimate causal link between mycobacterial infection and AIDS comes from the widespread geographical overlap of the two.

Worldwide, by conservative estimates, around one in three people are presently infected with *Mycobacteria tuberculosis* alone, or 1.7 billion people (WHO, 1995) and the very cities, in which up to 80% have tuberculosis, are the epicenters of AIDS. The last world AIDS conference in Barcelona admitted that 1/3 of all AIDS deaths were from diagnosed tuberculosis. (Naik, 2002)

Almost a million new cases of AIDS were estimated to be attributable to tuberculosis in 1995, and by the year 2000 there were probably 8 million co-infected people worldwide. (Quinn, 1999) Figures such as these make it unconvincing that AIDS ever surpassed tuberculosis as the leading cause of death in the world, especially in lieu of cross–reacting sera that opens up the question as to just how many cases attributed to HIV are in fact from tuberculosis or allied mycobacteria.

When the AIDS epidemic officially began in June 1981, allergist/immunologist Michael Gottlieb of UCLA, after first implicating cytomegalovirus (CMV), wrote *Ongoing AIDS Epidemic Could Be Product of Dual Pathogen Infection*, concluding that AIDS resulted from not one but two microbial infections. (Gottlieb, 1983) Unexpected in early AIDS autopsies was the surprisingly high proportion of difficult to diagnose *Mycobacterium avium-intracellulare* (Welch, 1984), in up to 55% (Kiehn, 1985) of American cases. But in Haitian and African AIDS patients, undoubtedly just as exposed to *Avium*, death by *Mycobacterium tuberculosis* predominated.

Most convincing evidence points to Gottlieb's hypothetical duel pathogens as being atypical mycobacteria such as *Avium* somehow getting into a human blood pool already harboring latent or active *Mycobacterium tuberculosis*. The "acquired" in Acquired Immune Deficiency Syndrome is *Mycobacteria avium* or a similar non-tuberculosis mycobacteria; "immune deficiency" but the result of a savage double attack on the immune system by an atypical mycobacterium (such as *M. avium*) and *M. tuberculosis*. *Avium* has, in the short space of 30 years,

Chapter 12/ LUCKY
L. Broxmeyer, M.D.

gone from relative obscurity to the leading infectious disease in U.S. and European AIDS, and there is no shortage in the literature for causes ranging from sexual transmission, (Damsker, 1985; De Capraris, 1984) to bestiality (Damsker, 1985; Katner, 1988), certain Voodoo practices, African ritualistic drinking of animal blood (Rapoza, 1986), and the medical or addicts use of shared needles (Roberts, 1989) to explain just how it could have been introduced and spread throughout the human blood pool, whether in Africa, the U.S., Europe or the rest of the world.

By the late 1960's, lymph nodes from 368 swine from Transvaal and Natal South Africa were examined and found to mostly contain *Mycobacteria avium complex* (MAC). (Kleeberg, 1969) Similar strains were then identified when attention shifted to humans in Africa in the early 1970's. (Kleeberg, 1975)

Only a few strains of MAC are found in human AIDS. (Kiehn, 1985) Notably these are also found in simian AIDS. (Henrickson, 1983) Weiszfeiler and Karczag (1973) succeeded in isolating 50 strains of Mycobactria, including MAC from 33 monkeys, a significant finding as millions of pre-AIDS Africans were vaccinated with an early polio vaccine attenuated in living monkey kidney tissue. Some see a correlation between where the bulk of polio vaccine was administered and the epicenters of AIDS. (Hooper, 1999) The Simiae-Avium (SAV) group of mycobacteria, which shares characteristics of both *M.avium* and *M. simiae*, by itself is entirely capable of causing a lethal AIDS infection. (MMWR, 2002)

Soil borne, MAC is found in cats, swine, and primates, all significant in early retroviral theories regarding AIDS.

The fertile soil upon which *Mycobacterium avium* and similar "atypical" mycobacteria plants AIDS is pre-existing TB, often latent, always immunosuppressive.

Chapter 12/ LUCKY
L. Broxmeyer, M.D.

Despite WHO estimates, Fox maintained that nearly half the world has TB (Fox, 1990) but others feel that number to be much greater.

Cantwell, who repeatedly found acid-fast forms in AIDS, felt it reasonable to assume that the initial immunosuppressive disease in that disease must also be present in many "healthy" people as studies indicate that some promiscuous but otherwise "healthy" gays were actually immunosuppressed to begin with. (Cantwell, 1983b)

Mycobacteria tuberculosis, both in its vast reservoir of seemingly well and human immune-killing potential, certainly fulfills this criteria. Papadopulos-Eleopulos (1995), reminds us that in African AIDS, "HIV infection" usually follows TB.

The first case of human disease due to *Mycobacterium avium-intracellulare* (MAC) was reported in a middle-aged Mesabi Range iron miner in 1943. His symptoms were pulmonary (Feldman, 1943) and until the emergence of AIDS, lung infection alone typified *Avium*, though differentiation between fowl or *Avium* tuberculosis and tuberculosis itself was at times nearly impossible. (Ortbals, 1978) The first reports of MAC in AIDS appeared in 1982 and Zakowski found it in 8 or 9 patients who died of AIDS at the UCLA Medical Center. (Zackowski, 1982)

Soon the devastatingly immunosuppressive potential of co-infection with *M. tuberculosis* and *M. avium* was shown. (Tsukamura, 1981) As already mentioned, this ability of mycobacteria to attack simultaneously is a recurrent theme in the literature, occurring over and over again. But in AIDS, it would bring on a combined immunosuppression the likes of which man had never had to deal with. The known ability for AIDS and TB to potentiate one another (Goldman, 1987) is a result of such double-pronged mycobacterial attack between

"AIDS", the atypical mycobacterial infection, and tuberculosis.

In such a scenario HIV is simply one of the L-forms of an atypical mycobacteria, in particular *M. avium* and until it is recognized as such no "retroviral" vaccine or cure will be possible.

In the U.S., on the surface, AIDS is characterized by the severe immunosuppression of *Mycobacteria avium* (MAC) and opportunistic infections like Kaposi's Sarcoma and *Pneumocystis carinii.* In Africa it's a wasting disease characteristically ending with death by *Mycobacteria tuberculosis.* HIV should cause the same disease where it from the same cause.

In <u>Disseminated *Mycobacterium avium* Infection Among HIV Infected Patients in Kenya,</u> Gilks approaches this most perplexing AIDS enigma in terms of the mycobacteria, addressing the apparent relative rarity of disseminated MAC in AIDS in Africa and the developing countries. (Gilks, 1995) That MAC exists in the African as well as the American environment (Von Reyn, 1993a) cannot be denied. Nor can the fact that African skin tests prove antibodies to MAC already in African blood. (Von Reyn, 1993b) Gilks acknowledges that AIDS victims in developing countries are probably dying of more virulent tubercular infections before they become immuno-suppressed enough to show *Avium.* Inderlied (1993) and O'Keefe (1996) agree.

Gilks mentions that AIDS patients in Africa, already infected with latent tuberculosis are more likely to reactivate this mycobacteria with catastrophic results before reaching the low CD4 level associated with clinical MAC. This, however, does not preclude that *Avium* or a similar non-tubercular mycobacteria, as causative, plants AIDS in the soil of previous tubercular infection, whether in Africa or elsewhere.

The full extent of drug-resistant TB in African countries is unknown but at least as prevalent as it is in New York, Haiti or the Ivory Coast. (Long, 1991) Frieden found 30% of resistant strains of tuberculosis in New York (Frieden, 1993) AIDS patients, but Shafer assured that with or without HIV, drug resistant tuberculosis was comparable. (Shafer, 1991)

How much of multi-drug resistant (MDR) TB is in fact a fusion with the atypical mycobacteria like MAC or SAV is an open question. Meanwhile, there hasn't been a new TB drug in 30 years. (Naik, 2002) For its part *Avium* (swine, or fowl tuberculosis) and the "atypical" mycobacteria in man have never had a truly satisfactory treatment. (Hafner, 1999) Whether this situation will change with novel strategies now in the pipeline (Broxmeyer & Sosnowska, 2002) remains to be seen.

Multi-drug-resistant strains always had the potential to render tuberculosis and *Avium* once again incurable infections. (De Cock, 1992) That this happened, and how new and virulent strains of mycobacteria found entry first into the human blood pool and then an enhanced portal of sexual transmission in the disease eventually called AIDS should come as a surprise to no one.

REFERENCES

PROLOGUE

al-Sumidaie AM, LeptsG Retrovirus in human breast cancer: detection of reverse transcriptase in human monocytes. *JR Coll Surg Edinb.* 33(3):151(3. 1988

Montagnier L *Vaincre le SIDA. Entretiens avec Pierre Bourget.* Paris, Editions Cana, 1986

Chapter 1. EPIDEMIC

MMWR Morb Mortal Wkly Rep 30:250(2. 1981

Chapter 2. CANCER STRUGGLES

Bittner JJ Some possible effects of nursing on the mammary gland tumor incidence of mice. *Sceince* 84:162. 1936

Diller I Donnelly Experiments with Mammalian Tumor Isolates. *Annals of the New York Academy of Sciences* 174(2):655-74. 1970

Duran-Reynals F Neoplastic Infection and Cancer. *American Journal of Medicine* 8(4):440-511. 1950

Ellermann V Bang O Experimentelle Leukamie bei Huhnern. *Zbt Bakt* 46:595-609. 1908

Francis DP Curran JW EssexM Epidemic acquired immune deficiency syndrome: Epidemilogic evidence for a transmissible agent. *J. Natl. Cancer Inst.* 71:1-4. 1983

Glover T Scott M A Study of the Rous Chicken Sarcoma No. 1 *Canada Lancet and Practicioner* 66(2):49-62. 1926

Klieneberger-Nobel E Origin, development and signifincance of L-forms in bacterial cultures. *J. Gen Microbiol* 3:434-442 1949

REFERENCES
L. Broxmeyer, M.D.

Livingston V A Specific Type of Organism Cultured from Malignancy: Bacteriology and Proposed Classification *Annals of the New York Academy of Sciences* 174:636-54 1970

Livingston V Cancer*: A New Breakthough.* Los Angeles. Nash Publishing. 1972

Martin W Medical *Heroes and Heretics.* The Devin Adair Company. Old Greenwich, Connecticut. 1977.

Mattman L Cell *Wall Deficient Forms – Stealth Pathogens.* CRC Press. Boca Raton. 1993.

Null G AIDS: A SECOND OPINION Townsend *Letter for Doctors and Patients June* 2000

Rous P A Sarcoma of the Fowl transmissible by an agent separable from the Tumor Cells. *J. Exp. Med.* 13:397-411.1911.

Roux E Sur les microbes dits inviibles *Bull. Instit Pasteur* 1:7–12, 49–56 1903

Seibert FB Feldman RL Morphological, Biological, and Immunological Studies on Isolates from Tumors and Leukemic Bloods. *New York Academy of Science* 174(2):690-728. 1970

Vallee H Carre H Nature infectieuse de l' anemie du chevale *C.R. Acad. Sci* Paris 139:331–33 1904

Wuerthele-Caspi V Alexander-Jackson E Cultural Properties and Pathogenicity of Certain Microorganisms Obtained from Various Proliferative and Neoplastic Diseases. *Amer J. Med. Sciences.* 220:638-646. 1950

Chapter 3. SHYH-CHING LO

Alexander-Jackson E A Specific Type of Microorganism Isolated from Animal and Human Cancer: Bacteriology of the Organism. *Growth* 18:37-51. 1954

REFERENCES
L. Broxmeyer, M.D.

Alexander-Jackson E Ultraviolet Spectrogramic Microscope Studies of Rous Sarcoma. *Annals of the New York Academy of Science.* 174(2):765. 1970

Burns DN Rohatgi PK Disseminated Mycobacterium fortuitum successfully treated with combination therapy including ciprofloxin. *Am Rev Respir Dis.* 142(2):468-470. 1990 Aug.

Gupta I Kocher J Mycobacterium haemophilum osteomyel itis in an AIDS patient. *NJ Med* 89(3):201-202. 1992 Mar.

Lemaitre M Guetard D Protective activity of tetracycline analogs against the cytopathic effect of the human immunodeficiency viruses in CEM cells. *Res Virol.* 141(1):5-16. 1990 Jan.

Livingston V Wuerthele-Caspe Livingston AF Some Cultural, Immunological and Biochemical Properties of *Progenitor Cryptocides.* Transactions of the New York Academy of Sciences. Series II. 36(6):569-82. 1974

Lo SC Isolation and identification of a novel virus from patients with AIDS. *Am J Trop Med Hyg* 35(4):657-6 1986 Jul.

Lo SC Dawson MS Identification of Mycoplasma incognitos infection in patients with AIDS; an immunohistochemical, in situ hybridization and ultrastructural study. *Am J. Trop Med Hyg* 41(5):601-16. 1989 Nov

Ostrom N Co-discoverer of AIDS virus says it may have microbial accomplice. *New York Native,* 1991 October 21

Parachini A New 'cure' for cancer stirs controversy. *Los Angeles Times.*1984, April 6

Roussel G Igual J. Clarithromycin with minocycline and clofazimne for Mycobacterium avium intracellulare complex lung disease in patients without the acquired immune deficiency syndrome. GETIM. Groups d'Etude et de Traitement des Infections a Mycobceries. *Int J Tuberc Lung Dis* 2(6):462-470. 1998 Jun.

AIDS: WHAT THE DISCOVERERS
OF HIV NEVER ADMITTED

REFERENCES
L. Broxmeyer, M.D.

Saillard C Carle P Genetic and serologic relatedness between Mycoplasma fermentans strains and a mycoplasma recently identified in tissures of AIDS and non-AIDS patients. *Res Virol* 141(3):385-95. 1990 May-Jun.

Seibert F Feldman R Morphological, Biological and Immunological Studies on Isolates from Tumors and Leukemic Bloods. *New York Academy of Science* 174(2):690-728. 1970

Tasaka S Urano T A case of Mycobacterium fortuitum pulmonary disease in a healthy young woman successfully treated with ciprofloxacin and doxycycline. *Kekkaku.* 70(1):31-35. 1995 Jan.

Tsukamura M Chemotherapy of lung disease due to Mycobacterium avium-Mycobacterium intracellulare complex by a combination of sulfadimethoxine, minocycline and Kitasamycin. *Kekkaku* 59(1):33-37. 1984 Jan.

Chapter 4. IN THE SEMEN OF MAN

Berthelsen, JD Economics of the avian TB problem in swine. *J. Am Vet Med Assoc* 164:307-8. 1974

Brunati J Tuberculosis of the penis; Surgical form-case. *Rev. de Chir* Paris 75:213-33. 1937

Centers for Disease Control (CDC) Immunodeficiency among female sexual partners of males with acquired immune deficiency syndrom (AIDS)-New York. *Morb Mortal Weekly Rep* 31:700-1. 1983

CDC Tuberculosis-United States, 1985-and the possible impact of human T-lymphotropic virus typeIII/lymphaden opathy associated virus infection. *Morb. Mortal Weekly Rep.* 35:74-6. 1986

CDC Diagnosis and management of mycobacterial infection and disease of persons with human immunodeficiency virus infection. *Ann Int Med* 106:254-6. 1987

REFERENCES
L. Broxmeyer, M.D.

Chakravarty SC Sircar DK Genital Tuberculosis in Males. Seminal Fluid Culture and Vaso-Seminal Vesiculography Studies. *J Indian Med Assoc.* 51(6):283-6. 1968 Sep 16

Chapman JS The atypical mycobacteria and human mycobacteriosis. New York. *Plenum.* 1977.

Damsker B Bottone EJ. *Mycobacterium avium-Mycobacterium intracellulare* from the Intestinal Tracts of Patients with the Acquired Immunodeficiency Syndrome: Concepts Regarding Acquisition and Pathogenesis. *J Infect Dis.* 151(1):179-81. 1985 Jan.

De Caprariis PJ Giron JA Mycobacterium avium-intracellulare infection and possible venereal transmission. *Ann Intern Med* 101(5):721. 1984

De Paepe ME Guerrieri C Waxman M Opportunistic infections of the testes in the Acquired Immunodeficiency Syndrome. *The Mt. Sinai Journ of Medicine.* 57(1):25-9. 1990 Jan

Giannacopoulos KC Hatzidaki EG Genital tuberculosis in a HIV infected woman. *Eur J Obstet Gynecol Reprod Biol* 80(2):227–9. 1998 Oct

Gondzik M Jasiewicz J Experimental study on the possibility of tuberculosis transmission by coitus. *Z Urol Nphrol* 72(12):911-14. 1979 Dec.

Heins Jr. HC Dennis EJ The possible role of smegma in carcinoma of the cervix. *Amer Journ Obstet Gynecol* 76:726–35 1958

Hellerstrom S *Acta Dermato-Venereologica.* 18 (4):465. 1937.

Hirschel, B in *HIV and AIDS.* Edited by Polsky and Clumeck. Mosby-Wolfe. London. 1999

Jara Rascon J Herranz Amo F Genito-urinary tuberculosis in acquired immunodeficiency syndrome. *Actas Urol Esp.*13(1):75-7. 1989 Jan.-Feb.

REFERENCES
L. Broxmeyer, M.D.

Jaisankar TJ Bhagath RG Penile Lupus Vulgaris. *International journal of dermatology.* 33(4):272-4. 1994

Jeyakumar W Ganesh R Papulonecrotic tuberculids of the glans penis: case report. *Genitourin Med* 64:130-2. 1988

Karlson AG The incidence of tuberculosis in animals in the U.S.A.. *Bulletin International Union Against Tuberculosis.* 40:61-3. 1968

Lal DN Sekhon GS Tuberculosis of the penis. *J. Indian Med Assoc* 56:316-18. 1971

Lattimer JK Colmore HP Transmission of Genital Tuberculosis From Husband to Wife Via The Semen. *Amer. Rev. Tuberc.* 69 (4):618-624. 1954 Apr.

Lewis EL Tuberculosis of the Penis. Report of 5 new cases and complete review of the literature. *J. Urol.* 56:737.1946

Lifson JD Reyes GR AIDS retrovirus induced cytopathology; giant cell formation and involvement of CD4 antigen. *Science* 232(4754):1123-7. 1986 May 30

Livingston, V. *Cancer: A New Breakthrough.* Los Angeles: Nash Publishing Company. 1972

Mavligit GM Talpaz M. Chronic immune stimulation by sperm alloantigens. Support for the hypothesis that spermatozoa induce immune dysregulation in homosexual males. *JAMA* 251(2):237-45. 1984 Jan.

Morrison JGL Fourie ED The papulonecrotic tuberculide: from Arthus reaction to lupus vulgaris. *Br. J. Dermatol* 91:263-70. 1974

Netter, FH Reproductive system. *The Ciba Collection of Medical Illustrations* West Caldwell, New Jersey 2:188. 1987

Nightingale SD Byrd LT Mycobacterium avium-intracellulare complex bacteremia in human immunodeficiency virus positive patients. *J. Infect Dis* 165:1082-5. 1992

Peer ET Genitourinary Transmission of Tuberculosis. *Amer Rev Tuberc* 75:153. 1957, Mar.

REFERENCES
L. Broxmeyer, M.D.

Piot P Quinn TC Acquired immunodeficiency syndrome in a heterosexual population in Zaire. *Lancet* 2:65-9. 1984

Popovic M Detection, isolation and continuous production of cytopathic retroviruses (HTLV-III) from patients with AIDS and pre-AIDS. *Science* 224(4648):497-500, 1984 May

Rolland R Schellekens L Genital tuberculosis, a forgotten disease? *Ned Tijdschr Geneeskd* 116(52):2377-8. 1972

Smith LH Wyngaarden JB *Cecil Textbook of Medicine* W.B. Saunders. Philadelphia. 1988

Van de Perre P Clumeck N. Female prostitutes: A risk group for infection with human T-cell lymphotropic virus type III. *Lancet* 2:524-526. 1985.

Van Voorhis BJ Martinez A Detection of human immunodeficiency virus type 1 in semen from seropositive men using culture and polymerase chain reaction deoxyribonucleic acid amplification techniques. *Fertil. Steril.* 55:588-594. 1991

Verneuil A Hypothesis on the origin of genital tuberculosis in the two sexes. *Gaz. Hebt d. Med* 25:225. 1883

Wilson-Jones E Winkelmann RK PapulonecroticTuberculo sis; a neglected disease in Western countries. *J. Am Acad Dermatol* 14:815-26. 1986

Wood B. An unusual cause of penile ulceration. *South African Med Journal* 79(1):284. 1991

Wyngaarden, JB Cecil Textbook of Medicine *W.B. Saunders Company.* Philadelphia. 19th Edition. 2: 1740. 1992

Chapter 5. CATS

Blaine DP Tuberculosis in the dog, cat and bird. *Vet Rec* 25:677. 1913

CDC Update: Acquired immunodeficiency syndrome (AIDS)-United States *Morb Mortal Weekly Rep* 32:465-7. 1983

REFERENCES
L. Broxmeyer, M.D.

Duesberg PH Retroviruses as Carcinogens and Pathogens: Expectations and Reality *Cancer Research* 47:1199-1220 1987, Mar.

Dorn CR Taylor D Cancer morbidity in dogs and cats from Alameda County. *J. Natl Cancer Instit.* 40:307-18. 1968.

Drolet R Disseminated tuberculosis caused by Mycobacterium avium in a cat. *J. Am Vet Med Assoc.* 189(10): 1336-7. 1986 Nov 15

Francis DP, Cotter SM Comparison of virus-positive and virus-negative cases of feline leukemia and lymphoma. *Cancer Research* 39:3899. 1979

Hix JW Jones TC Avian tubercle infection in the cat. *J Amer Vet Med Assoc* 138:641. 1961

Jarrett, WFH Crawford AM Leukemia in the cat: a virus-like particle associated with leukemia (lymphosarcoma) *Nature* 202:566-568. 1964

Jarrett O Laird HM Growth of feline leukaemia virus in human cells. *Nature* 224(225):1208-9. 1969 Dec 20

Jarrett O Laird HM Growth of feline leukemia virus in human, canine and porcine cells. *Bibl Haematol* 36:387-92. 1970

Jordan HL Disseminated Mycobacterium avium complex infection in three Siamese cats. *Am Vet Med Assoc* 204(1):90-3. 1994 Jan

Malik R Gabor L Subcutaneous granuloma caused by Mycobacterium avium complex infection in a cat. *Aust Vet J* 76(9):604-7. 1998 Sep

Miller MA Fales WH Inflammatory pseudotumor in a cat with cutaneous mycobacteriosis. *Vet Pathol* 36(2):161-3. 1999 Mar

Robin V Brion A Genital tuberculosis in a cat. *Rec Med Vet* 130:213. 1954

Rogerson P Jarrett W Epidemiological studies of feline leukemia virus infection. *Intl J. Cancer* 15:781-85. 1975

REFERENCES
L. Broxmeyer, M.D.

Snider WR Tuberculosis in Canine and Feline Populations. *Am Rev* of *Resp Disease* 104(6)877-87. 1971

Teas, J Could AIDS Agent Be a New Variant of African Swine Fever Virus? *Lancet* 1(8330):923. 1983 Apr 23

Chapter 6 .TRAGIC COST OF PREMATURE CONSENSUS

Barre-Sinoussi F Chermann JC Isolation of a T-lymphotropic retrovirus from a patient at risk for acquired immune deficiency syndrome (AIDS) *Science* 220:868-71. 1983

Fontes A Bemerkungen uber die Tuberkulose Infektion und ihr virus. *Mem Instit Oswaldo Crus* 2:141-146. 1910

Mellon and Fisher New Studies On The Filtrability Of Pure Cultures of the Tubercle Group of Microorganisms. *Journal of Infectious Disease* 51:117-28. 1932

Much H Die Variation des tuberkelbacillus in form and wirkung. *Beitr Klim Tuberk* 77:60-71. 1931

Chapter 7. THE RACE

Alexander-Jackson A Specific Type of Microorganism Isolated from Animal and Human Cancer: Bacteriology of the Organism. *Growth* 18:37-51. 1954

April MM Garelick JM Reverse transcriptase in situ polymerase chain readtion in atypical mycobacterial adenitis. *Arch Otolaryngol Head Neck Surg.* 122(11):1214-8. 1996 Nov

Bader JP Reproduction of RNA humor viruses *Comprehensive Virology* Plenum Press New York 4:253. 1975

Bess JW Microvesicles Are a Source of Contaminating Cellualr Proteins Found in Purified HIV-Preparations. *Virology* 230(1):134-44 1997 Mar

REFERENCES
L. Broxmeyer, M.D.

Cantwell AR Histologic Observation Of Variably Acid-Fast Coccoid Forms Suggestive of Cell Wall Deficient Bacteria in Hodgkin's Disease. A Report Of Four Cases. *Growth* 45:168-187. 1981

Gluschankof P Mondor I Cell Membrane Vesicles Are a Major Contaminant of Gradient Enriched Human Immunodeficiency Virus Type-1 Preparations. *Virology.* 230(1):125-33. 1997 Mar 31

Health Education AIDS Liaison (HEAL), HIV 101: 10 Scientific Reasons Why HIV Cannot Cause Aids. Toronto, 2001

Karpas A Unusual Virus Produced by Cultured Cells from a Patient with AIDS. Letter to Editor. *Mol. Biol. Med.* 1:457-459. 1983

Karpas A Maayan S Lack of antibodies to adult T cell leukemia virus and to AIDS virus in Israeli Falashas. *Nature.* 319:794. 1986

Lairmore MD Rosadio RH Ovine lentivirus lymphoid interstitial pneumonia. Rapid induction in neonatal lambs. *Am J. Path* 125:173-181. 1986

Livingston V Cancer: *A New Breakthough.* Los Angeles. Nash Publishing. 1972

Nambuya A Sewankambo N Tuberculosis lymphadenitis associated with human immunodeficiency virus (HIV) in Uganda. *J. Clin Pathol* 41:93-6. 1988

O'Hara CJ Groopman JE The ultrastructural and immunohistochemical demonstration of viral particles in lymph nodes from human immunodeficiency virus-related and non-human immunodeficiency virus-related lymphadenopathy syndromes. *Hum Pathol* 19(5):545-9. 1988 May

Seibert FB Feldmann FM Morphological, Biological, and Immunological Studies on Isolates from Tumors and Leukemic Blood. *Annals N.Y Acad of Sciences*: 174(3) 690-728. 1970

AIDS: WHAT THE DISCOVERERS
OF HIV NEVER ADMITTED

REFERENCES
L. Broxmeyer, M.D.

Voetberg A Lucas SB Tuberculosis or persistent generalized lymphadenopathy in HIV disease? *Lancet* 337:56-57. 1991

Watson E Hill LL Apojptosis in *Mycobacterium tuberculosis* infection in mice exhibiting varied immunopathology. *The Journal of Pathology* 190(2):211-220. 2000 3 Feb

---

Chapter 8. INVISIBLE VIRUS

Beral V Peterman TA Kaposi's sarcoma among persons with AIDS: a sexually transmitted infection? *Lancet* 335:123-128. 1990

Cantwell Jr. AR Lawson JW Necroscopic findings of pleomorphism, variably acid-fast bacteria in a fatal case of Kaposi's sarcoma. *J Dermatol Surg Oncology* 7:923-930. 1981a

Cantwell Jr. AR Bacteriologic investigation and histologic observations of variably acid-fast bacteria in three cases of Kaposi's sarcoma. *Growth* 45:79-89. 1981b

Cantwell Jr. AR Variable acid-fast bacteria in vivo in a case of reactive lymph node hyperplasia occurring in a young male homosexual. *Growth* 46: 331-336. 1982

Cantwell AR Jr Necroscopic findings of variably acid-fast bacteria in a fatal case of acquired immunodeficiency syndrome and Kaposi's sarcoma. *Growth* 47: 129-134. 1983

Cantwell Jr. AR Mycobacterium avium-intracellulare infection and immunoblastic sarcoma in a fatal case of AIDS. *Growth* 50:32-40. 1986

CDC. Centers for Disease Control Task Force on Kaposi's Sarcoma and Opportunistic Infections. Epidemiologic Aspects of the current outbreak of Kaposi's sarcoma and opportunistic infections. *N Eng J. Med* 306:248-52. 1982

Chen YJ, Shieh PP. Orificial tuberculosis and Kaposi's sarcoma in an HIV-negative individual. *Clin Exp Dermatol* 25(5):393-7 2000 July

REFERENCES
L. Broxmeyer, M.D.

Cohen RJ, Samoszuk MK, Busch D et al Occult infection with M. intracellulare in bone marrow biopsy specimens from patient with AIDS. *New Engl Jourl of Medic* 308:1475-1476. 1983

Croxson TS, Ebanks D Atypical mycobacteria and Kaposi's sarcoma in the same biopsy specimens. *New Engl J. Med* 308: 1476. 1983

Moore JP Ho DD HIV-negative AIDS. *Lancet* 340:475. 1992

Tsukamura M Mizuno S Occurrence of *Mycobacterium tuberculosis* and strains of the *Mycobacterium avium-M intracellulare* complex together in the sputum of patients with pulmonary tuberculosis. *Tubercle* 62:43-46. 1981

Zakowski P, Fligiel S Disseminated Mycobacterium avium-intercellulare infection in homosexual men dying of acquired immunodeficiency. *JAMA* 248: 2980-2982. 1982

Chapter 9. SMOKE AND MIRRORS

Clavel F Guetard D Isolation of a new human retrovirus from West African patients with AIDS. *Science.* 233:343-46. 1986

DeCock KM Tuberculosis and HIV infection in Sub-Saharan Africa *JAMA* 268:12. 1992 Sept 23/30

Iseman MD Evolution of drug resistant tuberculosis: A tale of two species. *Proc Nat Acad Sci* USA Vol 91:2428-29. 1994, Mar

John JJ Kaur A Tuberculosis and HIV infection. *Lancet* 342(2):676. 1993

Kashala O Infection with human immunodeficiency virus type 1 (HIV-1) and human T-cell lymphotropic viruses among leprosy patients and contacts: correlation between HIV-1 cross-reactivity and antibodies to lipoarabinomannan.*J. Infect Dis* 169(2):296-304. 1994 Feb

REFERENCES
L. Broxmeyer, M.D.

Kemper CA Meng TC Treatment of *Mycobacterium avium* complex bacteremia in AIDS with a four-drug oral regimine: rifampin, ethambutol, clofazimine and ciprofloxacin. *Ann. Intern. Med.* 116:466-472. 1992

Lowell, AM. *Tuberculosis in the world.* DHEW Publication No. CDC 76-8317. Washington DC: US Government Printing Office. 3-27. 1976

Modilevsky T Sattler FR Mycobacterial disease in patients with human immunodeficiency virus infection. *Arch. Intern Med.* 149:2201-2205. 1989

Serwadda D Slim disease: a new disease in Uganda and its association with HTLV-III infection. *Lancet* 2(8460):849-52. 1985 Oct 19

Stead WW Asim K D Epidemiologic and Host Factors in *Tuberculosis.* Praeger Monographs in Infectious Disease Vol 2. Praeger. New York. 1983

Veronese FM Characterization of gp41 as the transmembrane protein coded by the HTLV-III/LAV envelope gene. *Science* 229:1402. 1985

Chapter 10. AMBIGUOUS SLAUGHTER

Armstrong JA Hart PD A Response of cultured macrophages to *Mycobacterium tuberculosis*, with observations on fusion of lysosomes and phagosomes *J. Exp Med* 134:713–740 1971

Armstong JA Hart PD Phagosome–lysosome interactions in cultured macrophages infected with virulent tubercle bacilli. Reversal of the usual nonfusion pattern and observations on bacterial survival *Journal of Experimental Medicine* 142:1–16. 1975

REFERENCES
L. Broxmeyer, M.D.

Bermudez LE Parker A Growth within macrophages increases the efficiency of *Mycobacterium avium* to invade other macrophages by complement receptor independent pathway. *Infect Immun* 65:1916-25. 1997

Bermudez LE Parker A Apoptosis of *Mycobacterium avium*-infected macrophages is mediated by both tumour necrosis factor (TNF) and Fas, and involves the activation of caspases. Clin Exp. Immunology. 116:94-99. 1999

Bultmann BD Flad HD Disseminatred mycobacterial histiocytosis due to M. fortuitum associated with helper T-lymphocyte immune deficiency. *Virchow's Arch* 395:217-25. 1982

Chaouchi N Arvanitakis L Characterization of transforming growth factor-B1 induced apoptosis in normal human B cells and lymphoma B cell lines. *Oncogene* 11:1615-22. 1995

Detels R, English, PA, Patterns of CD4+ Cell Changes After HIV-1 Infection Indicate the Existence of a Codeterminant of AIDS. *J. Acquir. Immune Defic. Syndr.* 1:390-395. 1988

Dlugovitzky D Luchesi S Circulating immune complexes in patients with advanced tuberculosis and their association with autoantibodies and reduced CD4+ lymphocytes. *Braz J Med Biol Res* 28(3):331-5. 1995 Mar

Donahoe RM Bueso-Ramos C Mechanistic Implications of the Findings That Opiates and Other Drugs of Abuse Moderate T-cell Surface Receptors and Antigenic Markers. *Ann. N. Y. Acad. Sci.* 496:711-721. 1987

Duesberg PH Aids epidemiology: inconsistencies with human immunodeficiency virus and with infectious disease. *Proc Natnl Acad Sci* 88:1575-9. 1991

Duesberg PH AIDS acquired by drug consumption and other noncontiguous risk factors. *Pharmac Ther 55:201-277.* 1992

Fratazzi C Arbeit RD Macrophage apoptosis in mycobacterial infections. *J. Leukoc Biol* 66(5):763-4. 1999 Nov

REFERENCES
L. Broxmeyer, M.D.

Gangadharam PR Pratt PF In vitro response of murine alveolar and peritoneal macrophages to Mycobacterium intracellulare *Am Rev Respir Dis* 128(6):1044–7 1983 Dec

Gilks CF Richard JB Disseminated Mycobacterium avium Infection Among HIV Infected Patients in Kenya. *J. Acquired Immune Defic Synd Hum Retroviral* 8(2):195-8. 1995 Feb 1

Hirsch CS Toossi Z Apoptosis and T Cell Hyporesponsiveness in Pulmonary Tuberculosis. *The J of Infect Dis.* 179:945-953. 1999

Ho DD Rota TR Infection of monocyte-macrophages by human T-lymphotropic virus type III. *J. Clin. Invest* 77:1712-15. 1986

Jaworowski A Crowe SM Does HIV cause depletion of CD4+ T cells in vivo by the induction of apoptosis? *Immunol Cell Biol.* 77(1):90-8. 1999 Feb

John JJ Kaur A Tuberculosis and HIV infection. *Lancet* 342(2):676. 1993

Lamoureux G Davignon L Is prior mycobacterial infection a common predisposing factor to AIDS in Haitians and Africans? *Ann Inst Pasteur Immunol* 138(4):521-9 1987 Jul-Aug

Lemaitre M Guetard D Protective activity of tetracycline analogs against the cytopathic effect of the human immunodeficiency viruses in CEM cells. *Res Virol* 141(1):5-16. 1990 Jan.-Feb

Levy J Mysteries of HIV-challenges for therapy and prevention. *Nature* 333:519-22. 1988

McDonald I, Wang H Transforming growth facor B1 cooperates with anti-immunoglobulin for the induction of aptosis in group I (biopsy-like) Burkitt lymphoma cell lines. *Blood* 87:1147-54. 1996

REFERENCES
L. Broxmeyer, M.D.

McDonough KA Kress Y Pathogenesis of tuberculosis: interaction of Mycobacterium tuberculosis with macrophages - published erratum appears in Infect Immun 1993 Sep;61(9):4021–4) *Infect Immun* 61(7):2763–2773. 1993 July

Molloy A Laochumroonvorapong P Apoptosis, but not necrosis, of infected monocytes is coupled with killing of intracellular bacillus Calmette-Guerin. *J. Exp Med* 180:1499-509. 1994

Mudaki Y Perriens JH Spectrum of immunodeficiency in HIV-1-infected patients with pulmonary tuberculosis in Zaire. *Lancet* 342(8864):143-6. 1993 July 17

Novick DM Brown DJC Influence of Sexual Preference and Chronic Hepatitis B Virus Infection on T Lymphocyte Subsets, Natural Killer Activity, and Suppressor *Hepatol.* 3:363-370. 1986

Ohtomo K Wang S Secondary infections of AIDS autopsy cases in Japan with special emphasis on Mycobacterium avium-intracellulare complex infection. *Tohoku J Exp Med* 192(2):99-109. 2000 Oct

Papadopulos-Eleopulos E Turner VE A Critical Analysis of the HIV-T4-Cell AIDS hypothesis. *Genetica* 95:5-24. 1995

Pieters J Entry and survival of pathogenic mycobacteria in macrophages. *Microbes and Infection.* 3(3):249–55. 2001 Mar

Reeve PA Tuberculosis & HIV infection. *Lancet* 342(2):676. 1993

Rhoades ER Ullrich HJ How to establish a lasting relationship with your host: lessons learned from Mycobacterium spp. *Immunol Cell Biol* 78(4):301–10. 2000 Aug

Rojas M Olivier M TNF-alpha and IL-10 modulate the induction of apoptosis by virulent Mycobacterium tuberculosis in murine macrophages. *J. Immunol* 162(10): 6122-31. 1999 May 15

REFERENCES
L. Broxmeyer, M.D.

Teitelbaum R Cammer M Mycobacterial infection of macrophages results in membrane–permeable phagosomes. *Proc Natl Acad Sci* 96(26): 15190–5. 1999 Dec 21

Tsukamura M Mizuno S Occurrence of *Mycobacterium tuberculosis* and strains of the *Mycobacterium avium-M. intracellulare* complex together in the sputum of patients with pulmonary tuberculosis. *Tubercle* 62:43-46. 1981

WHO: Statement of AIDS and tuberculosis. Geneva. WHO. 1989

Chapter 11. VIRAL MIRAGE

Bermudez LE Parker A Apoptosis of *Mycobacterium Avium* infected macrophages is mediated by both tumor necrosis factor (TNF) and Fas and involves the activation of caspases. *Clin Exp Immunol* 116:94-99. 1999

Centers for Disease Control. Weekly Surveillance Report. October 20, 1986

Conlan MG Interview with David Rasnick Ph.D.: On Columbia's AIDS Conference and the Nature of Science Zenger's *News Magazine, San* Diego. 1998 Jan.

Dubos R Dubos J The *White Plaugue* Rutgers University Press New Brunswick. 1952

John JJ Kaur A Tuberculosis and HIV infection. *Lancet* 342(2):676. 1993

Johnson C The PCR to Prove HIV Infection. Viral Load and Why They Can't Be Used. Continuum (London) 4:33-37. 1996

Jones JL Hanson DL HIV-associated tuberculosis in the era of highly active antiretroviral therapy. The Adult/Asolescent Sprectrum of HIV Disease Group. *Int J Tuberc Lung Dis* 4(11):1026-31. 2000 Nov.

REFERENCES
L. Broxmeyer, M.D.

Kaplan, JE Hanson MS Epidemiology of human immunodeficiency virus–associated opportunistic infections in the United States in the era of highly active anti–retroviral therapy. *Clin Infect Dis.* 30 Suppl1:S5–14 2000

Lyles RH Tang AM Virologic, immunologic, and immune activation markers as predictors of HIV-associated weight loss prior to AIDS. Multicenter AIDS Cohort Study. *J. Acquir Immune Defic Syndr* 22(4):386-94. 1999 Dec. 1

Regush N The *Virus Within.* New York Plume. 2001 March

Chapter 12. LUCKY

Bisburg E Central Nervous System Tuberculosis with the Acquired Immunodeficiency Syndrome and its Related Complex. *Annals of Internal Medicine* 105:210-13. 1986

Blattner W Gallo RC HIV causes AIDS Science 241(4865):515-6. 1988 Jul 29, 241

Broxmeyer L Sosnowska D Miltner E Chacon O Wagner D McGarvey J Barletta RG Bermudez LE Killing of *Mycobacterium avium* and *Mycobacterium tuberculosis* by a Mycobacteriophage Delivered by a Nonvirulent Mycobacterium: A Model for Phage Therapy of Intracellular Bacterial Pathogens. *The Journ of Infectious Diseases* 186(8):1155–60. 2002 Oct 15

Cantwell Jr. Ar *Aids: The Mystery and The Solution.* Aries Rising Press. Los Angeles. 1983b

Damsker B Bottone EJ *Mycobacterium avium-Mycobacterium intracellulare* from the Intestinal Tracts of Patients with the Acquired Immunodeficiency Syndrome: Concepts Regarding Acquisition and Pathogenesis. *J Infect Dis.* 151(1):179-81. 1985 Jan

De Caprariis PJ Giron JA Mycobacterium avium-intracellulare infection and possible venereal transmission. *Ann Intern Med* 101(5):721. 1984

REFERENCES
L. Broxmeyer, M.D.

DeCock K, Benoit S Tuberculosis and HIV infection in sub-Saharen Africa regardless of HIV status *JAMA* Vol 268(12). 1992 Sep

Elliot JL Hoppes WL The acquired immunodeficiency sydrome and Mycobacterium avium-intracellulare in a patient with hemophilia. *Ann. Int. Med.* 98:290-293. 1983

Feldman WH Davies HE An unusual mycobacterium isolate from sputum of a man suffering from pulmonary disease of long duration. *Am. Rev. Tuberc* 48:272-290. 1943

Fox JL TB: A Grim Disease of Numbers. ASM News. Vol 56:363-64 1990

Frieden TR Sterling T The emergence of drug-resistant tuberculosis in New York City. *New Engl J. Med* 328:521-26. 1993

Gilks CF Richard JB Disseminated *Mycobacterium avium* Infection among HIV Infected Patients in Kenya. *J. Acquired Immune Defic Synd Hum Retroviral* 8(2):195-8. 1995 Feb. 1

Goldman KP AIDS and tuberculosis. *British Med J.* 295:511-12. 1987

Gondzik M Jasiewicz J Experimental study on the possibility of tuberculosis transmission by coitus. *Z Urol Nphrol* 72(12):911-14. 1979 Dec

Gottlieb MS Ongoing AIDS epidemic could be product of dual pathogen infection. *Skin and Allergy News* 14: 1983, Jan

Hafner R Inderlied DM Correlation of quatitative bone marrow and blood cultures in AIDS patients with disseminated *Mycobacterium avium* complex infection. *J. Infect Dis* 180:438–47. 1999

Hagmar B Kutti J Disseminated infection caused by *Mycobacterium kansasii*. Report of a case and brief review of the literature. *Acta Med Scand* 186:93-9. 1969

REFERENCES
L. Broxmeyer, M.D.

Hazra R Robson CD Lymphadenitis due to non- tuberculosis mycobacteria in children: presentation and response to therapy. *Clin Infect Dis* 28(1):123-9. 1999 Jan

Henrickson RV Maul DH Epidemic of acquired immunodeficiency in rhesus monkeys. *Lancet* 1:388-390. 1983

Hooper, E The *River A Journey to the Source of HIV and AIDS* Little Brown and Company Boston. 1999

Inderlied CB Kemper CA The *Mycobacterium avium* Complex. Clinical Microbiology Reviews 266-310 1993. Jul

Jawahar MS Scrofula revisited: an update on the diagnosis and management of tuberculosis of superficial lymph nodes. *Indian J. Pediatrics* 67(2):528-33. 2000 Feb

Katner HP Origin of AIDS. *Journal of the National Medical Association.* 80:262. 1988

Kiehn TE Edwards FF Infections caused by *Mycobacterium avium* complex in immunocompromised patients: diagnosis by blood culture and fecal examination, antimicrobial susceptibility tests, and morphological and seroagglutination characteristics. *J. Clinical* Microbiol. 21 168-173. 1985

Kleeberg HH Nel EE Porcine mycobacterial lymphadenits *J.S. Afr. Vet Med Assoc.* 40:233–250 1969

Kleeberg HH Gartig D Experience with sample surveys among African tribes and their annual risk of infection. 23rd International Tuberculosis Conference, Mexico City, Sept. 22–26, 1975

Lamoureux G Davignon L Is prior mycobacterial infection a common predisposing factor to AIDS in Haitians and Africans? *Ann Inst Pasteur Immunol* 138(4):521-9. 1987 Jul.-Aug

Long R Impact of human immunodeficiency virus type 1 on tuberculosis in rural Haiti *Am Rev Respir Dis* 143:69-73. 1991

AIDS: WHAT THE DISCOVERERS OF HIV NEVER ADMITTED

REFERENCES
L. Broxmeyer, M.D.

MMWR Disseminated Infection with Simiae-Avium Group Mycobacteria in Persons with AIDS – Thailand and Malawi, 1997 Centers for Disease Control and Prevention (CDC) 51-23):501–502. 2002

Naik G Agency to Unveil AaJoint Assault on TB and HIV. *Wall Street Journal.* July 9, 2002

O'Keefe EA Wood R AIDS in Africa *Scand J. Gastroenterol Suppl* 220:147-52. 1996

Ortbals DW Marr JJ A comparative study of tuberculosis and other mycobacterial infections and their associations with malignancy. *Am Rev Respir Dis* 117:39-45. 1978

Papadopulos-Eleopulos E Turner VF AIDS in Africa: distinguishing fact and fiction. *World Journal of Microbiology & Biotechnology.* 11:135-143. 1995

Perrone C Mycobacterial infections in AIDS *Rev Prat* 45(6):729-32. 1995 Mar

Peterman TA Stoneburner RL Risk of human immunodeficiency virus transmission from heterosexual adults with transfusion-associated infections *J Am Med Assoc.* 259:53. 1988

Quinn TC HIV-AIDS-Related Problems in Developing Countries from *HIV and AIDS,* a section taken from *Infectious Diseases by Armstrong and Cohen.* Mosby-Wolfe. London. 1999

Rapoza N An AIDS experts grim message. *American Medical News.* 1986, December 5

Roberts DJ Tuberculosis and HIV infection in Africa 298(1):751. 1989

Shafer,RWChirgwin KDHIV prevalence, immunosuppression and drug resistance in patients with tuberculosis in an area endemic for AIDS. *AIDS* 5:399-405. 1991

Schonell ME Crofton JW Disseminated infection with *Mycobacterium avium. Tubercle* 49:12-30. 1968

REFERENCES
L. Broxmeyer, M.D.

Terrones R de Alarcon A Mixed adenitis caused by Mycobacterium avium complex and Mycobacterium tuberculosis complex in patients with HIV infection. *Enferm Infecc Microbiol Clin* 15(4):225-6. 1997 Apr

Tsukamura M Mizuno S Occurrence of *Mycobacterium tuberculosis* and strains of the *Mycobacterium avium-M. intracellulare* complex together in the sputum of patients with pulmonary tuberculosis. *Tubercle* 62:43-46. 1981

Von Reyn CF, Waddel RD. Isolation of *Mycobacterium avium* complex from water in the United States, England, Zaire and Kenya. *J. Clin Microbiology* 31:3227-30. 1993a

Von Reyn CF Barber TW. Evidence of previous infection with *M. avium* among healthy subjects: an international study of dominant mycobacterial skin test reactions. *J. Infect Dis* 168:1553-8. 1993b

Weiszfeiler JG Karczag E Study of mycobacteria strains belonging to the Avian-Intracellular Group Isolated From Monkeys. *Ann Soc Beig Med Trop* 53(4):315-20. 1973

Welch K Finkbeiner W Autopsy findings in the acquired immune deficiency syndrome. JAMA 252 1152-1159. 1984

Williams G Stretton TB Leonard JC AIDS in 1959? *Lancet* 2:1136. 1983

World Health Organization (WHO). *WHO report on the tuberculosis epidemic, 1995.* Geneva. World Health Organization. 1995

Youmans GP Tuberculosis WB Saunders Comp Philadelphia: 318-325. 1979

Zakowski P Fligiel S Disseminated *Mycobacterium avium-intracellulare* infection in homosexual men dying of acquired immunodeficiency *JAMA* 248:2980-2. 1982

INDEX

A

acid-fast6, 26, 30, 32, 33, 34, 67
Actinomycetales 6
African Swine Flu Virus 21
AIDS .. i, iii, iv, v, 1, 2, 3, 8, 9, 11, 13, 17, 18, 19, 20, 21, 22, 23, 24, 25, 27, 28, 29, 30, 32, 33, 34, 35, 36, 37, 39, 40, 41, 42, 45, 46, 47, 48, 49, 50, 51, 52, 53, 54, 55, 56, 58, 59, 60, 61, 62, 63, 65, 66, 67, 68, 69, 70, 71, 72, 73, 74, 75, 76, 77, 78
Alexander-Jackson, Dr. Eleanor . 10, 30, 58, 59, 65
apoptosis 39, 70, 71, 72
avium-intracellulare's 48

B

bacteriocidal 47
Barre-Sinoussi, Dr. F. . 25, 65
bestialily 19, 53
bone marrow biopsy ... 34, 68
Breast Cancer .... v, 6, 57

C

Cancroids 16
Cantwell Jr, Dr. Alan .. 30, 32, 33, 34, 54, 66, 67, 74
cat leukemia 3, 21
CD4 cell count 39, 40
CD4 lymphocytes 27, 41
Cell-wall deficient bacteria .. 8

Centers for Disease Control 1, 60, 67, 73, 77
Co-factor theory 9
consumption 38, 70
contraceptives 18
Curran, Dr. James 2, 5, 57
Cytomegalovirus 2

D

Damsker, Dr. Beca 18, 19, 20, 53, 61, 74
disseminated tuberculosis .36
drug addicts 1
drug resistant tuberculosis56, 68
Duesberg, Dr. Peter ... 22, 28, 39, 41, 64, 70

E

electron microscope 6, 49, 50
enlarged lymph nodes .29, 34
epidemic tuberculosis 35
Essex, Dr. Myron ... 5, 21, 22, 23

F

factor VIII 1, 50
Factor VIII blood transfusions 50
Feline Leukemic Virus *see* FeLV 22
FeLV 21, 22
fowl or swine tuberculosis *see Mycobacterium avian-intracellulare* 18
Francis, Dr. Donald .. 2, 5, 22, 57, 64

G

Gallo, Dr. Robert ..11, 21, 22, 23, 25, 27, 28, 29, 30, 45, 74
genital tuberculosis15, 18, 63
giant cells 17
global emergency..............37
Gottlieb, Dr. Michael....52, 75

H

heterosexual....35, 37, 63, 77
Highly Active Antiretroviral Therapy –(HAART) 46
HIVi, iii, iv, v, 8, 9, 11, 13, 17, 18, 28, 29, 30, 31, 32, 33, 35, 36, 37, 38, 39, 40, 41, 45, 46, 47, 48, 49, 50, 51, 52, 54, 55, 56, 61, 65, 66, 67, 68, 70, 71, 72, 73, 74, 75, 76, 77, 78
Ho, Dr. David....................45
HTLV1 ....22, 23, 29
HTLV-3...............................28
human growth hormone 11

I

immune system ..1, 8, 40, 48, 51, 52

J

Jarrett, Dr. William.............21

K

Karpas, Dr. Abraham 29
Klieneberger, Dr E.........8, 57

L

Lattimer, Dr. John........14, 50
LAV..................25, 27, 28, 69
lentivirus 5, 66

L-forms..8, 11, 26, 30, 55, 57
lipoara-binomannan-LAM .36
Livingston, Dr. Virginia........6
Lo, Dr. Shyh-Ching 9
lymphadenopathy 25, 60, 66, 67
lymphadenopathy XE "lymphadenopathy" associated virus see LAV 60
lymphogranuloma inguinale 16
lysosome.....................42, 69
lysozyme 42

M

MAC..........14, 53, 54, 55, 56
macrophage kill.................43
macrophages .40, 41, 42, 69, 70, 71, 72, 73
MAI 14, 48
Montagnier, Dr. Luc ...iii, 8, 9, 24, 25
Mullis, Dr. Kary..................45
Mycobacterium avium see Mycobacterium avium–intracellulare .. 13, 18, 19, 33, 50, 52, 53, 54, 55, 59, 60, 61, 62, 64, 67, 68, 69, 70, 71, 72, 73, 74, 75, 76, 77, 78
Mycobacterium fortuitum .59, 60
Mycobacterium gordonae 33
Mycobacterium tuberculosis.... 15, 37, 40, 50, 52, 67, 68, 69, 72, 73, 74, 78
Mycoplasma..........49, 59, 60

N

National Cancer Act............ 7
non-tuberculosis
    mycobacteria 52

O

oncoviruses......................... 7
opportunistic infections 2, 32,
    55, 67, 74

P

Papadopulos-Eleopulos, Dr.
    E.................. 39, 54, 72, 77
Pasteur Institute, The 5, 24,
    25
Peer, Dr. Edgar T.............. 15
penile ulcerations.............. 17
PGL-Persistent Generalized
    Lymphadenopathy)....... 36
phagosome...................... 42
phenolic glycolipid 36
Pleomorphic.................. 8, 30
Pneumocystis carinii..... 1, 32
polio vaccine 53
Polymerase Chain Reactors-
    PCR 13, 45
protease inhibitors 47, 48

R

**reactive lymph node
    hyperplasia**............ 34, 67
retroviral particles 29
retroviral theory of AIDS ... 32

retrovirus ....v, 2, 6, 8, 10, 11,
    21, 23, 24, 25, 26, 27, 28,
    29, 37, 46, 49, 62, 65, 68
reverse transcriptase....7, 27,
    57
RNA tumor viruses 30
Rous Sarcoma.............10, 59
Rous, Dr. Peyton 6, 7, 10, 11,
    57, 58, 59

S

See Arc.............................37
Slim disease 69
slow virus..........................28
Syphilis 16, 18, 35

T

TB *see Mycobacterium
    tuberculosis* .....iii, iv, 5, 14,
    17, 26, 35, 37, 40, 41, 42,
    47, 51, 53, 54, 56, 60, 75,
    77, 78
TB virus 26
T-cells lymphocytes
    see CD4 Lymphocytes.... 2
Teas, Dr. Jane...................21
Temin, Dr. Howard 7
tubercle bacilli. 14, 15, 17, 69
tuberculosis of the penis ..16,
    18
tuberculosis ulcers.............16

V

viral load 45, 46